Unani

*

The Science of
Graeco-Arabic
Medicine

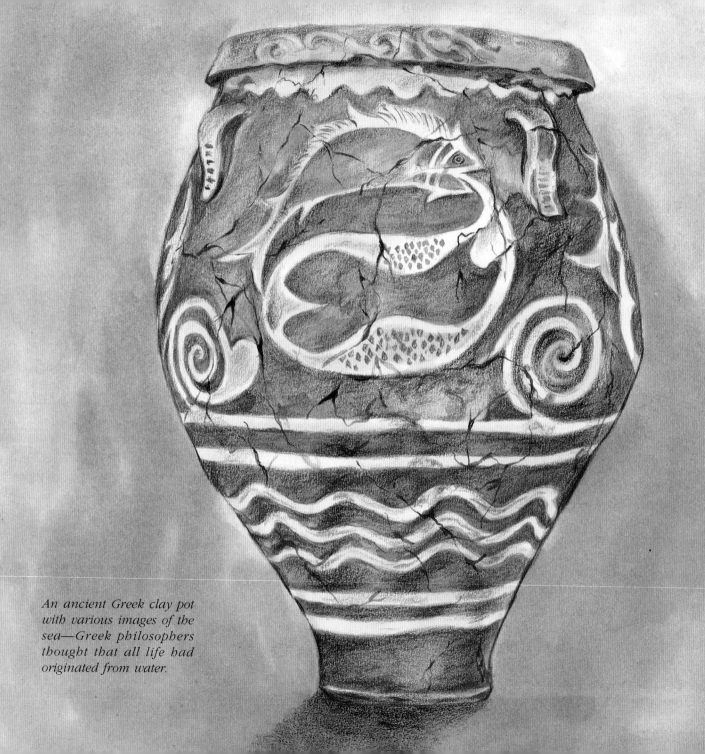

An ancient Greek clay pot with various images of the sea—Greek philosophers thought that all life had originated from water.

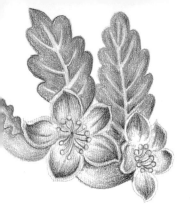
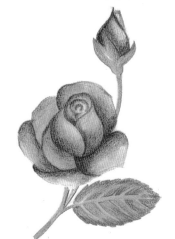

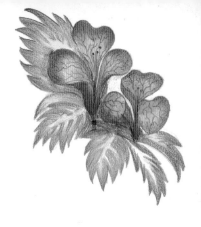
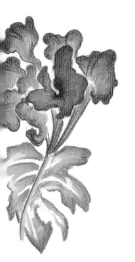
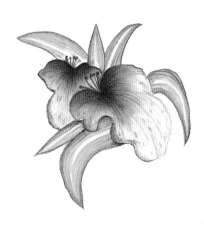

Unani

*

The Science of

Graeco-Arabic
Medicine

*

PROF. JAMIL AHMAD
HAKIM ASHHAR QADEER

Lustre Press
Roli Books

Dedication
————— ✳ —————

This book is dedicated to Padamshree Hakim Abdul Hameed, one of the greatest Unani physicians of present times and the founder of Hamdard University, New Delhi. He helped to keep Unani medicine alive in India when it was almost dying after Independence. At 87, he remains actively involved in developing this form of treatment. Recently, he was acclaimed as the Scholar of the Time in an award ceremony held in Iran.

Foreword
———— ✳ ————

The system of Unani medicine is based on the basic principles of diagnosis and treatment of diseases laid down by Greek philosophers and physicians— Hippocrates (460-370 BC) and Galen (AD 131-210). The system was later adopted by the Arabs, who by the 10th century AD, had enriched and advanced it through scientific methods and inclusion of what was best in the contemporary system of traditional medicine in the Arab world. The contributions of Rhazes, Avicenna and others are significant. Their writings are still held to be authoritative and referred to by Unani physicians. The Unani system is now known as Graeco-Arabic medicine. The Arabs introduced this system in India in the 12th century where it was further enriched by the drugs and remedies from the indigenous system. After the downfall of the Mughal empire, state patronage to Unani medicine was withdrawn. Inspite of this, Unani medicine survived in India because of the efforts of scholars genuinely interested in keeping it alive. Hakim Abdul Hameed is one such scholar who has been working ceaselessly towards reviving and advancing the system.

Unani medicine emphasises the power of self-preservation called *Quwat-e-Mudabirrah (medicatrix naturae)* in order to maintain the correct humoural balance in the human body—a pre-requisite for health.

At the time of the origin of Unani medicine in Greece or during the period of its development in the Arab world and India, humankind was not exposed to environmental stress and pollution as today. Present-day scholars and practitioners find it very difficult to undertake research and develop appropriate remedies in the changing and polluted biosphere. However, Unani medicine seems to be steadily gaining popularity even in the Western world as the drugs prescribed by this system are made up of natural products and have no toxic side-effects.

This book by Prof. Jamil Ahmad and Hakim Ashhar Qadeer covers all the features of the Unani art of healing and science. It contains five chapters which include an introduction, the concept of the human body, maintenance of health, concept of diseases, laws of treatment and home remedies.

I hope the readers will find this book not only interesting but useful as well. I congratulate the authors for their efforts in popularising Unani medicine through this book.

Prof. Alauddin Ahmad
Vice-chancellor
Jamia Hamdard
New Delhi

First Published 1998
© **Lustre Press Pvt. Ltd. 1998**
M-75, Greater Kailash-II Market,
New Delhi-110 048, INDIA
Phones: (011) 6442271, 6462782, 6460886
Fax: (011) 6467185

ISBN: 81-7436-052-2

Authors:
Jamil Ahmad
Hakim Ashhar Qadeer

Illustrations:
Ajoy Kumar Biswas
Conceived & Designed at
ROLI CAD CENTRE

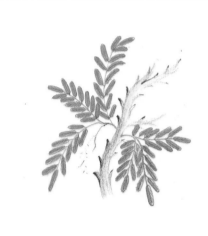

Text Editor:
Arundhati Roy Chowdhury

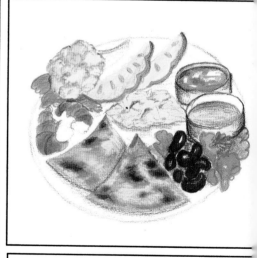

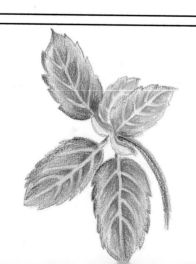

Printed and bound by
Star Standard Industries Pte. Ltd.
Singapore

Foreword
5

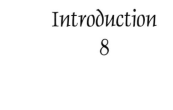

Introduction
8

The Concept of
the Body
20

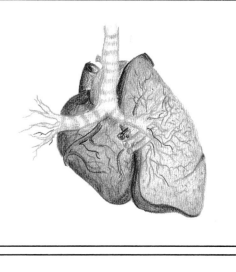

Maintenance
of Health
30

Concept of Diseases
& their Cure
38

Home Remedies
54
Glossary
82

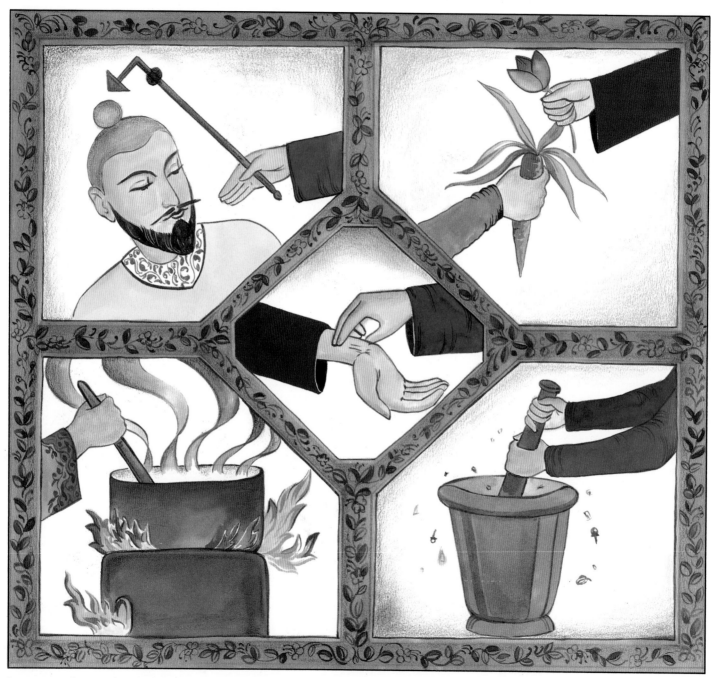

Some typical procedures of diagnosis, treatment and cure used in Unani medicine.

An Introduction to
Unani Medicine

———— ✳ ————

Greek Medicine or Tibb-e-Unani

Avicenna (Ibn Sina in Arabic, AD 980-1037), the ancient Unani physician with the most far-reaching impact on the Islamic and the Western world, defined Unani medicine as the science by which we learn the various states of the body in health and when not in health, and the means by which health is likely to be lost, and when lost, is likely to be restored.

Unani medicine, like any other form of medical science, strives to find the best possible ways by which

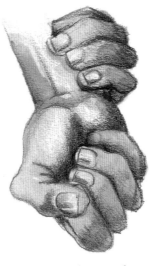

Nabz *or pulse. Reading a patient's pulse is one of the most widely practised methods of Unani diagnosis.*

a person can lead a healthy life with the least sickness. According to the Unani discipline, the human body is composed of seven natural and basic components which are responsible for the maintenance of health. The loss of any one of these basic components or alteration in their physical state could lead to disease or even to death.

The logic behind maintaining good health is based on the concepts of hygiene or *hifzan-e-sehat* and the six essential causes to maintain health or *asbab-e-sittah zaruriah*. These causes are explained briefly in the chapter titled Maintenance of Health.

The causes of diseases and their classification according to symptoms and modes of manifestation are stated in the chapter Concept of Diseases. This chapter gives the reader an understanding of pathogenesis or the onset of a disease.

For the diagnosis of a disease, the most important aspects are pulse or *nabz,* urine or *boul* and foecal matter or *baraz.* As far as the cure of diseases is concerned, all diseases are treated on four lines. The first is regimental therapy or *ilaj-bit-tadbir.* The special techniques used in this therapy are massage or *dalak,* exercise or *riyazat* and steam bath or *hammam* . The second line of therapy is known as diet-o-therapy or *ilaj-bil-ghiza* in which alterations in the quality and quantity of the patient's diet are suggested. In this, either the patient is asked to restrict his or her diet or a balanced diet is suggested for malnourished patients. Sometimes, the patient is even asked to forego food altogether.

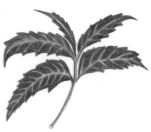

Neem *or the margosa tree is well-known for its medicinal powers* .

The third line of therapy is pharmacotherapy or *ilaj-bid-dawa.* In this kind of treatment, natural drugs i.e. drugs of natural origin are used. They may be of plant, animal or mineral origin. The methods of preparing the drugs and the form in which they are to be taken are explained later.

Surgery or *jarahat* is the fourth line of treatment. Some special surgical methods used in Unani medicine are venesection or *fasd,* cupping or *hijamat,* leeching or *taleeque* and diathermy or cauterization or *amal-e-kai.*

Every system of medicine is based on a definite anatomical and physiological concept of a human being. The science of Unani medicine considers the human body a natural living compound and all its activities like construction, destruction and their management performed according to natural laws. The power which administers all these activities is known as *tabiat* which can be roughly translated as physic or the art of healing. This power is given to every individual by nature. If this power is strong, the body functions smoothly; if it weakens, one falls ill. What it needs for its sustenance are a natural atmosphere and resources to survive. Anything unnatural, either from the atmosphere or resources can weaken this power. For example, a polluted atmosphere or impurities in food and water affect its strength which in turn leads to disease.

In case of disease, the Unani physician strives to activate this power as it is the natural healer of the body. The physician either suggests ways of purifying the atmosphere and the natural resources or prescribes a remedy. The remedy however, always attempts to be as close to nature as possible. For example, if a small wound occurs, it heals without any effort; but if the wound is big, only then the physician sutures the wound. Suturing is an unnatural process and means a

Nuqrah *and* tila *or silver and gold respectively. Mineral drugs used as general tonics for over-all bodily well-being.*

forceful intrusion into the body. This violation of nature can very well lead to other complications.

Unani medicine is distinct from other branches of medicine as the drugs it uses are natural in their sources and forms. It emphasizes on retaining natural compounds which belong to the human body and hence prescribes only natural remedies.

Unani medicine believes that diseases can be kept at bay by the use of clean and fresh water, breathing clean and fresh air, and consuming clean and fresh food. Likewise, a balance should be maintained between the mind and the body so that the metabolic processes can take place easily and the body waste evacuated.

Historical Background

Since the very beginning of life, there is death and disease. Hence, the history of medicine is as old as the

11

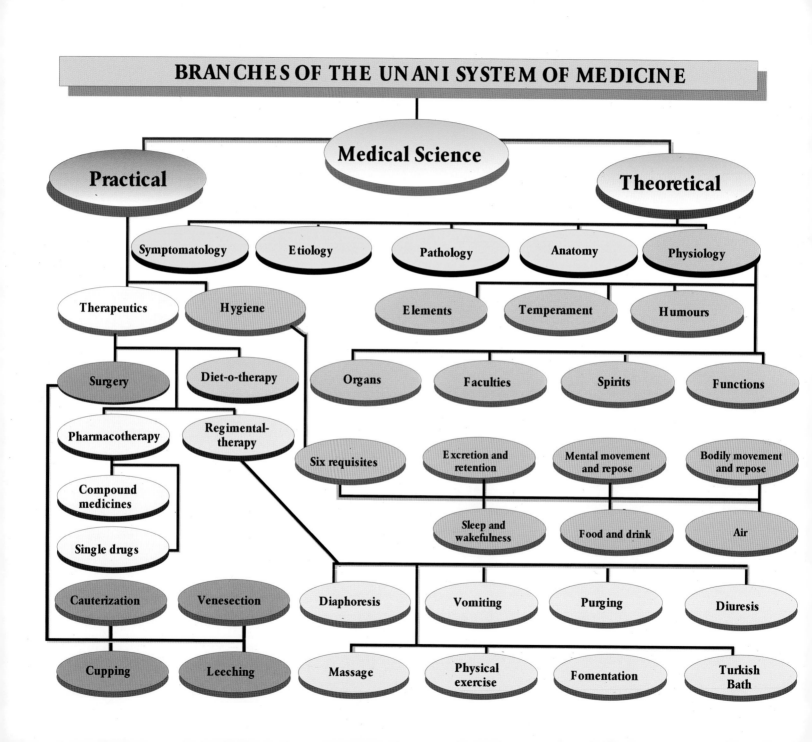

history of civilization. The study of medicine flourished in all ancient civilizations. Some ancient medical systems are Misri tibb (Egyptian medicine), Hindi tibb (Indian medicine), Chini tibb (Chinese medicine) and Unani tibb (Greek medicine). The Unani art of healing is still a living system and is practised with a lot of zeal and fervour by Unani physicians.

The theory and practice of Unani medicine as a natural process of treatment originated in Greece (Unan in Arabic). The Greeks had accumulated a wealth of pragmatic information on maintaining good health over the centuries. Their philosophers had developed rational theories and methods of treatment. In the fifth century BC, Greek medicine was given form and recognition as a scientific system by Hippocrates or Buqarat (460-377 BC) who is considered the father of Unani medicine.

Hippocrates freed medicine from the realm of superstition and magic.

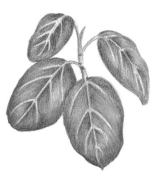

Bargad *or the banyan tree. Each part of this tree is used for medicinal purposes.*

He established the theoretical framework of Unani medicine basing it on the theory of humours. According to him, the human body contains four humours; blood or *dam*, phlegm or *balgham*, yellow bile or *safra* and black bile or *sauda*. As long as these humours are combined in the right proportions, a person is healthy, when they are not, disease sets in.

After Hippocrates, a number of Greek scholars improved and expanded the scope of the system. The Greek physician, Galen or Jalinoos (AD 131-210) was probably the most influential and prolific. Thorough in the existing medical knowledge of the time, he based his philosophy and theories on experimental evidence.

Aristotle (384-322 BC) had said, "Nature does nothing without a purpose." Galen agreed and felt that since nature always had a clear purpose, an organ too must have a specific function. To affirm this, he defined the structure and functions

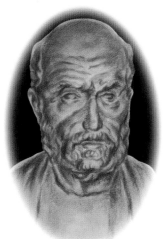

Hippocrates
460-377 BC

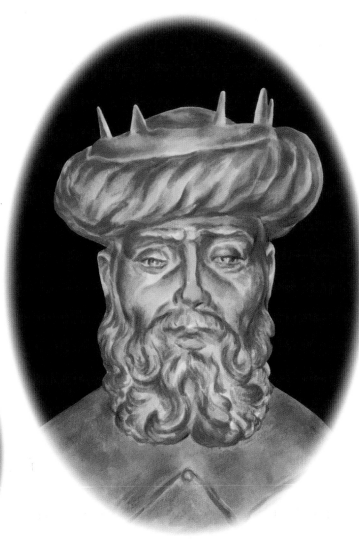

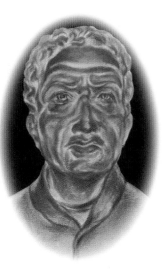

Galen
AD 131-210

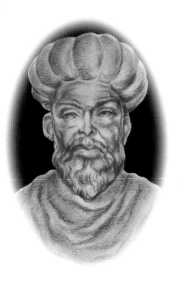

Avicenna
AD 980-1037

Rhazes
AD 865-925

Zahravi
AD 946

of all body organs and established a concept of anatomy as well as physiology of the human body.

After a long journey through Greece, Rome and Iran, Unani medicine came to the Arab world. This was the golden period of the Arab civilization known as the Abbasit Caliphate (AD 749-1258) or *Khilafat-e-abbasia*. The Arab scholars of the time converted almost all the Greek, Roman and Latin medical and scientific work into Arabic. The city of Baghdad, which was the capital of King Haroon Rashid (AD 786-809), came to be known as the great seat of knowledge as it became a major centre of learning, renowned for its efforts in the field of medicine. Many centres of academic advancement such as the Bait-ul-Hikamat were developed. The government patronised the sciences by recognising and rewarding scholars who translated other medical works into Arabic. And gradually an entire

Kibreet *or sulphur, a mineral drug, mostly used as a disinfectant.*

system of medical science, Graeco-Arabic medicine or Unani, was born.

Arab scholars wrote valuable treatises on various aspects of Unani medicine. During the same period, the scope of Unani medicine was improved and expanded by the theories of Ayurvedic medicine which reached the Arab countries. Many renowned *vaidyas* (Ayurvedic physicians) were invited to Baghdad and several Ayurvedic treatises like *Susruta Samhita* were translated into Arabic.

Rhazes (AD 865-925) was a famous and almost legendary healer of the Arab world. He said, "All that is written in a book is worth much less than the experience of a wise doctor." His most celebrated work is *Al Havi Libre Continents* which encompasses all the practical and clinical concepts of Unani medicine. In his time, Unani medicine was at its peak and became so advanced that many hospitals and dispensaries were

15

opened for treating common people.

Abul Quasim Zahravi was another important contributor in the development of Unani medicine. Abdul Quasim was born in the city of Zahra near Cordoba in Andalusia in AD 946. The city of Cordoba was a centre of classical learning. When he grew up, Abul Qasim became a surgeon in the Royal Hospital of Cordoba. By that time, the Arabs had developed surgery to a high degree of sophistication. Operations on the thorax and other viscera had become very common.

The most significant work of Zahravi is *Al-Tasreef,* a book on surgery. This book is still considered a complete and comprehensive treatise on surgery with pictures of surgical instruments invented by Zahravi himself which were amongst the finest of the time. Zahravi was also the first to introduce a new posture for women in labour, now known as the Walcher position. Zahravi's works were referred to as

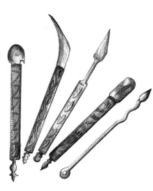

Some Unani surgical instruments invented by Zahravi.

documentary proof of Unani medicine in all European medical colleges for many centuries. Many modern surgeons allude to Zahravi in their works.

The concepts of Unani medicine were refined in the tenth and eleventh centuries by Ibn Sina (AD 980-1037). Born in Bukhara, he studied philosophy and medicine and travelled very widely. He gathered all the ideas of Unani medicine scattered in the various contemporary schools of scholasticism as he felt these ideas were dominated by pedantry which made them difficult to understand and less practical in treating diseases. He freed the theories from these shackles and reformulated them from a clinical point of view in his book *Al Qanon Fit Tibb,* latinised as *The Canon of Medicine.* The *Qanon* has also been translated into Uzbek, Turkish, Hebrew and Urdu. It was used as an authoritative medical text all over the world including Europe and the Arab

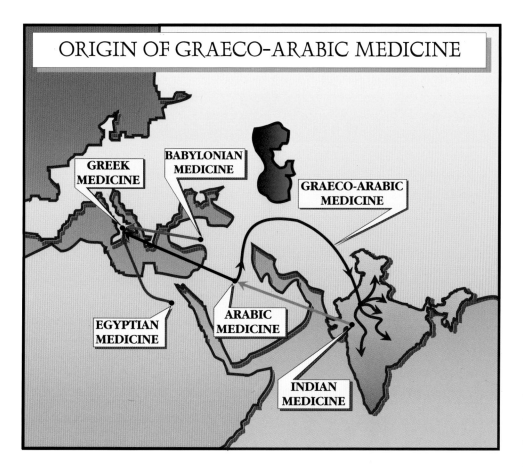

ORIGIN OF GRAECO-ARABIC MEDICINE

GREEK MEDICINE

BABYLONIAN MEDICINE

GRAECO-ARABIC MEDICINE

EGYPTIAN MEDICINE

ARABIC MEDICINE

INDIAN MEDICINE

the Arab region. The Arabs nurtured and developed it extensively.

Introduction in India

Between the 6th and 5th centuries BC, while the Indian system of medicine or Ayurveda was reigning supreme in the East, the Greeks were busy advancing medical knowledge in the West. Then came a time in the 13-14th century AD when Arab scholars introduced the Unani system in India.

world for almost eight centuries. Even today, it is considered an encyclopedia of Unani medicine.

Thus Unani medicine developed as a complete and unique system of medicine mostly during its reign in

In the 14th century AD when the Mongols ravaged the Persian and central Asian cities like Shiraz, Tabrez and Alam, scholars and physicians of Unani medicine fled to

India. The Delhi sultans: the Khiljis, the Tughlaqs and the Mughal emperors provided state patronage to the scholars and even enrolled some as state employees and court physicians. Between the 13th and 17th centuries, Unani medicine was at its peak in India. The most eminent amongst those who made valuable contributions to this system in this period was Hakim Ali Gilani. Hakim Gilani was a brilliant mathematician and engineer who came to India from Iran (Gilan in Arabic) during the reign of Akbar the Great (1556-1605) and soon after became personal physician to the emperor. He was a fervent scholar and an intelligent physician which soon earned him the title: "Galen of the Age" (*Jalinoos-e-Zaman*). He compiled an extensive commentary on Ibn Sina's *Al Qanon* in Arabic.

Development

The Unani physicians who fled from Persia to settle in India subjected Indian drugs to clinical trials and as a result of their experiments, added numerous drugs to their own system, thus further enriching its treasures. The system found immediate favour with the Indian people and soon spread all over the country and continued to hold an unchallenged place for a long time even after the downfall of the Mughal empire.

During the British rule in India, Unani medicine suffered. Its development was hampered due to the withdrawal of government support. But since the masses had complete faith in the system, it continued to be practised. It was mainly due to the efforts of ancient families of *hakims* (Unani physicians), who wanted to keep the tradition alive, like the Sharief family in Delhi, and the Azizi family in Lucknow during the late 18th and early 19th centuries and the Nizam of Hyderabad that Unani medicine survived in the British period.

At present, the Unani system is well established in Asia. The major

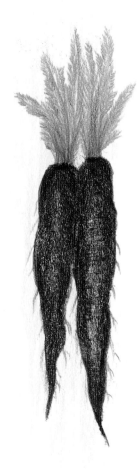

Gazar or carrot. A widely eaten seasonal vegetable whose seeds have medicinal properties.

centres of Unani medicine are India, Pakistan, Bangladesh and Sri Lanka where there are recognised Unani practitioners, hospitals, educational and research institutions.

An outstanding physician and scholar of Unani medicine, Hakim Ajmal Khan (1864-1926) championed the cause of the system in India. The Hindustan Dawakhana and the Ayurvedic and Unani

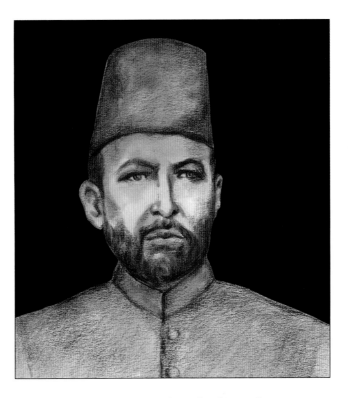

Hakim Ajmal Khan (1864-1926)

Tibbia College in Delhi are examples of his immense contribution to the two systems of medicine.

In India, the leading institution for the study and practice of Unani medicine is the Hamdard University in New Delhi. The university is perhaps the only institute in Asia which conducts complex research in Unani pharmacology, pharmacognosy and pharmacy.

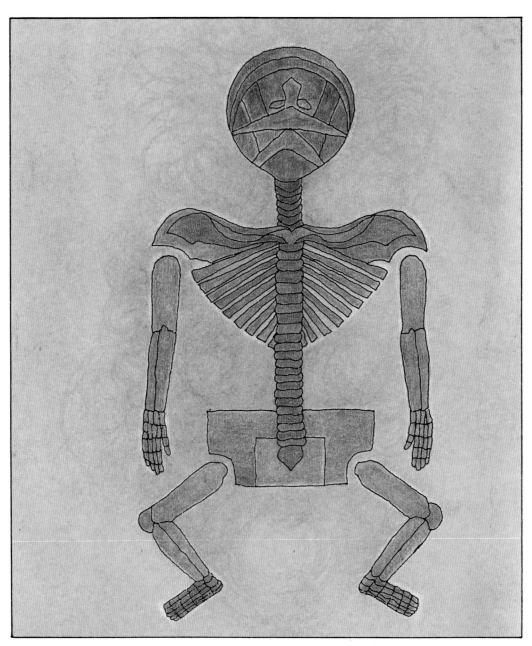

The skeletal system, as visualised by the Unani *system. Drawing based on a late 14th century illustrated manuscript.*

The Concept of the Body

———— ✳ ————

The concept of the body under Unani physiology is known as *umure tabaiyah* and is based on seven natural principles. These principles start from the basic units of the body i.e. its constituent elements or *arkan* and end with body functions or *afal-e-badam*.

According to the theories of Unani medicine, *tabiat* is a mysterious power all living beings possess to maintain good health. *Tabiat* not only ensures all body functions are performed smoothly but fights against disease during illness.

The concept of *tabiat* was laid down by Hippocrates. He said, "Nature heals, the physician is only

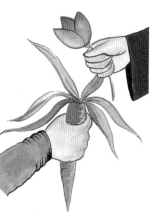

All Unani drugs have to originate purely from nature.

nature's assistant." And that is why he advised physicians to abide by and follow the power of *tabiat* and not antagonise it. After Hippocrates, many other scholars too stressed on the importance of the concept of *tabiat.*

They said that *tabiat* works in two ways: it administers body functions involuntarily, it performs actions suitable to the body. The strength of this power is inversely proportional to the duration of a disease.

The philosophy behind the ancient theories *of tabiat* is that it is a natural power responsible for keeping the body healthy. If this power weakens, a physician has to be consulted. As long as this power remains strong, the healing process takes place on its own. This is evident from the fact that minor diseases like wounds heal and close up without any treatment, many painful conditions subside after sleep and without the aid of medicines.

The Seven Natural Principles

Elements

Among the seven natural principles, the first is that of elements or *arkan*. These are simple individual substances which provide the primary components for a compound. They cannot be further dissolved into simpler entities. Thus, all types of matter found in nature are formed by the combination of these substances. The quality of a compound, physical as well as

Primary Elements
ELEMENTS AND PROPERTIES
Nar or **Fire** -Hot and dry (*har* and *yabis*).
Hawa or **Air**-Hot and wet (*har* and *ratab*).
Ma or **Water**- Cold and wet (*barid* and *ratab*).
Arz or **Earth**-Cold and dry (*barid* and *yabis*) .

chemical, depends on the specific nature of each constituting element. In other words, the element is the basic unit of a compound.

According to the ancient precepts of Unani theory there are four primary elements: fire or *nar*, air or *hawah*, water or *ma* and earth or *arz*. These elements are the basic building blocks of all substances in nature including the human body. This theory of the four primary elements was widely accepted by Hippocrates, Aristotle, Galen, Avicenna and all other subsequent scholars.

These four elements also determine the four states of matter. Air stands for the gaseous state, water stands for the liquid state, earth stands for the solid state and fire stands for matter which has been transformed into heat. Each of these elements have their own properties as shown in the chart above.

Each element contains two properties in which one is active and one passive. For example, in fire, heat is an active property which has the productive capacity while dryness is a passive property and remains dormant. Two active properties can never be found in an element i.e. an element cannot be simultaneously hot and cold.

Every element has a certain temperament or *mizaj* which makes every compound differ in nature as far as chemical and physical states are concerned. Therefore, physically three types of matter are found: solid, liquid and gaseous and chemically there are hot, wet, cold, and dry states of matter. The human body contains all types of matter and their properties will be discussed later.

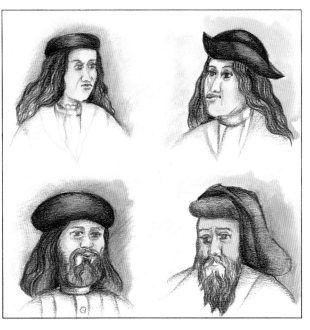

The four temperamental personalites (AD 1500). Top left: melancholic man, top right: sanguine man, bottom right: phlegmatic, bottom left: choleric. (From: The Guild Book of the Barber-surgeons of York, *British Museum).*

Temperament

The second principle is temperament or *mizaj.* Temperament can be defined as a new state which is the result of the actions and reactions between the contrary qualities present in different elements. The resultant uniform state which emerges after the combination of the properties of more than one element is called temperament.

On the basis of this intermixture, two types of compounds are formed. If two or more elements are simply mixed and their individual properties are maintained as before, it is a simple intermixture. For example, when sugar and water are mixed, the resultant syrup has the qualities of both. If the elements are changed altogether and the new compound formed has completely new properties, it is called a factual combination or *imtizaj haquiqui*.

On the basis of the proportion of elements in a compound, temperament is further classified as:

- *Equal temperament:* When the contrary qualities of elements present in a compound are equal in quantity and perfectly balanced according to the required properties and functions of that compound, it is known as equal temperament or *mizaj-e-mutadil*. Hence, when we say a body has an equal temperament, it means that it performs its functions smoothly and is in a homeostatic state.
- *Unequal temperament:* When the

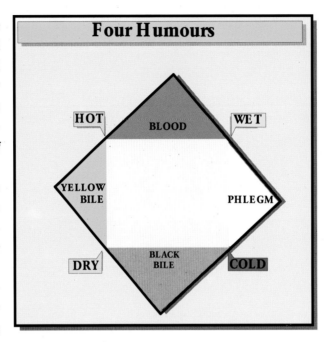

Four Humours

HOT   BLOOD   WET

YELLOW BILE   PHLEGM

DRY   BLACK BILE   COLD

opposite qualities of the elements in a compound are quantitatively unequal and unbalanced, its unequal temperament or *mizaj-e-ghair mutadil* causes abnormal body func-tions and leads to disease. This unbalanced temperament is further divided into two kinds:

i) *Simple:* In the simple unbalanced or *mufrad* temperament, a single quality predominates more than others. This may be heat, cold, dryness or moisture.

ii) *Compound:* In compound or *murakkab* temperament, two qualities out of the four are more dominant than others. These may be hot-dry, hot-moist, cold-dry or cold-moist.

Humours

The ancient Unani scholars based their medical system on the basis of the theory of humours which combined both physiology and pathology. According to them, in the human body, there are three types of matter as far as physical state is concerned i.e. liquid, solid and gaseous. The solid parts are known as organs or *azah*, liquid parts are known as humours or *akhlat* and the gaseous as pneuma or *rooh*.

The body fluids, which are humours, are further sub-divided into four types: blood *(dam)*, phlegm (*balgham*), yellow bile (*safra*) and black bile (*sauda*). Blood is regarded as a mixture of all four kinds of humours. Because of the predominance of *dam* and the mixture's strong red colour, it is called *dam*. The temperament of blood is hot and moist.

Phlegm is a colourless fluid. The temperament of phlegm is cold and moist.

Yellow bile is a yellow fluid in the body. It comes after blood and phlegm in order of importance and is temperamentally hot and dry.

The heart and blood vessels where all body humours are present.

Black bile is black in colour and the least important amongst all the humours. It has a cold and dry temperament.

This humoural concept was suggested by Hippocrates in his book *Tabiatul Insan*. This theory suggests that every person is supposed to have a unique humoural constitution which represents his or her state of health. If an imbalance in quality or quantity of humours occurs, it leads to sickness.

If each human being has a particular constitution of humours, then on the basis of this constitution, people can be categorised under four basic temperaments. The temperament of an individual is determined by the humour which is most predominant.

Human temperament then is determined by the proportion in which the four humours are found in an individual's body. The four types of temperament are sanguine temperament or *damwi mizaj* in which blood predominates, bilious temperament or *safrawi mizaj* in which yellow bile predominates, phlegmatic temperament or *balghami mizaj* where phlegm is the dominating factor and melancholic temperament or *saudawi mizaj* where black bile is all-important. Signs and symptoms of each temperament will be discussed in a later chapter.

The concept of humours and their importance has held credibility in medical science since medieval times. The term "humours" is applicable to all kinds of fluids found in the body, irrespective of their colour, location, quantity and composition. Therefore, cellular fluids, tissue fluids and vascular fluids all come under the term humours.

All body fluids have a normal range, quality and composition which is known as their phycological value. When this phycological value is disturbed, disease sets in.

Imbalance in the quantity of humours causes diseases which occur

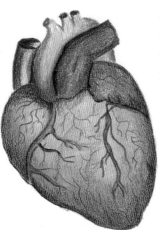

The qualb *or heart. Source of vital power.*

due to excessive loss or extra accumulation of fluids either in the whole body or in a part of the body. Diseases like malnutrition, vitamin deficiency and hormonal disturbances are results of such an imbalance.

Body Organs

As mentioned earlier, three types of matter are found in the body and the solid part is made up of organs or *azah*. These organs are derived primarily from the coarser and more concrete particles of the humours.

Organs are classified into two kinds as far as structure is concerned: simple and compound. A simple organ is defined as an organ in which the smallest part exactly resembles the whole. A simple organ is therefore completely homogeneous in structure. Thus a tiny piece of flesh is still flesh and a branch of nerve still resembles a nerve.

Therefore the simple organs are: flesh (*lahem*), bone *(azm)*, nerve *(asb)*, cartilage *(ghuzruf)*, tendon *(wat'r)*, membrane (*ghishah*), fat (*shahem*), artery (*shiryan*), vein (*warid*). Some scholars also include marrow (*mukhkh*), nail (*zufur*) and hair (*shar*) in the list of simple organs.

Compound organs are those which are heterogeneous and are composed of many simple organs, like the face, the feet and so on. Organs are also classified according to their functions. There are some vital organs or *azah-e-raisah* on which the primary and essential powers of the body depend, most important of which is the power to live.

The main or vital organs which are important for the survival of an individual are four:

- *The heart:* According to Aristotle, the heart or *qalb* is the first organ which is formed in the life of an embryo. It is the source of vital power or innate heat. It is served by blood vessels which transport oxygen from the heart to various body organs.
- *The brain:* Hippocrates differs from Aristotle by saying that the brain

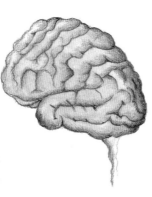

The dimagh *or brain. The seat where all sensations originate.*

or *dimagh* is the first organ to be formed in the embryo. It is the seat of all powers as far as sensations and movements are concerned. It is served by a network of nerves which carry instructions sent by it to the body organs.

- *The liver:* The liver or *kabid* is an organ from which all nutritive and vegetative powers originate. The liver contains vessels which emerge from it to carry nutritive material to all other organs of the body.
- *The testes:* The testes or *khisya* is a specifically male organ which is concerned with reproduction. It ensures the propagation of a species.

According to Unani theories, organs can be classified on the basis of their origin also. Some scholars believe that the simple organs originate from the seed of the male (semen or *mani*) when the foetus is being formed and are known as *azah-e-manwiah*. Later the mother's blood nourishes the embryo and takes part in the formation of organs which are known as *azah-e-damwiah*.

Another group of scholars say that all simple organs except the flesh and fat originate from the semen in the zygotic stage. The flesh originates from the denser portion of the blood and heat coagulates it while fat arises from the greasy portion of the blood and cold coagulates it. Therefore fat melts when heat is applied.

Faculty

All work performed by the body require a certain power and an ability to do which are assigned by factors called faculties or *quwat*. In other words the phenomenon by which all life functions are manifested is *quwat*. There are different types of body functions and there are various kinds of faculties. The faculties provide the basis for these different bodily functions, and are to be distinguished from the functions themselves. Faculties give

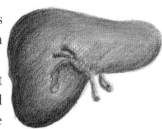

The kabid *or liver. The organ which controls body nutrition.*

rise to functions but every function requires its own special faculty. A faculty actually means an entire system or group of organs which are perfectly synchronised and take part in a particular metabolic function. The term "digestive faculty" of an individual therefore means the participation of the liver, blood vessels, intestines and other associated organs in the process of digestion.

Thus, faculties may be defined as those natural and specialized powers which are furnished to a human body for the performance of its specific functions, and which become the cause for the performance of specific functions by the organs of the body for the preservation of the individual as well as species. Faculties are divided into three major divisions:

- Natural faculty or *quwat-e-tabia*.
- Mental faculty or *quwat-e-nafsaniya*.
- Vital or physical faculty or *quwat-e-haiwaniya*.

28

Pneuma

According to Galen, air is composed of various substances; the most important of them, the one on which life depends, is pneuma or vital air or *rooh*. Modern scientists have discovered this essential element to be oxygen.

Unani medicine says that after an individual inhales, the inhaled air is purified in the lungs i.e. pneuma is separated from it, it is sent to the heart. Hence, Galen considered the heart to be the source of innate heat. Since ancient times Unani physicians have believed that the chief function of the heart is to pump pneuma (oxygenated blood) to the different organs of the body.

Functions

The term functions or *afal* came to be used in Unani medicine to

The heart and the lungs. Organs whose combined action generates pneuma or vital air.

designate the normal or special performance of a part of the body. Unani scholars say that some of the bodily functions are carried out by a single faculty (like attraction, propulsion, retention and digestion). These are therefore called simple functions. Some other functions are carried out by a group of faculties acting in unison. The faculty of attraction, i.e. the first gesture towards food when a person is hungry and the body longs for food by sending internal signals, which is achieved by longitudinal fibres at the orifice of the stomach and esophagus, and the faculty which conducts the propulsion of the food to the stomach which is carried out by the voluntary muscles of the throat, help in swallowing food. Thus, the complete act of eating is one of the compound functions of the body.

29

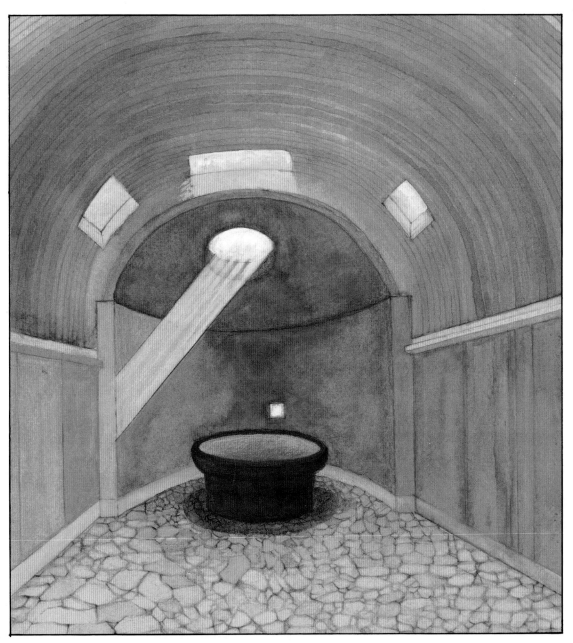

The hamam, *one of the traditional regimens of Unani medicine, is a room where the atmosphere is kept warm by hot air to give a patient steam fomentation.*

Maintenance of Health

✳

Unani medicine believes in preventive measures rather than curative. There are six basic factors which are essential for the maintenance of good health. By obeying the rules determined by these factors the body becomes strong and less prone to diseases. These factors, called *asbab-e-sittah zaruriah* or six essential causes, are:

- Air or *hawah*.
- Food and drink or *makool-o-mashroob* .
- Body movement and repose or *harkat-wa-sukoon badania*.
- Mental movement and repose or *harkat-wa-sukoon nafsania*.
- Sleeping habits or *naum-o-yaqzah* .

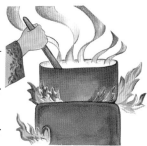

A classical Unani method of sterilization to remove impurities.

- Retention and evacuation *ehtibas-o-istafraagh*.

Air

Fresh and clean air is essential for good health. Polluted air weakens the body and makes it more vulnerable to diseases. The process of respiration can be performed better if the air is fresh as polluted air affects the respiratory organs and has an adverse effect on them.

There are many factors which make the air impure; humidity being one of them. Therefore, it is better to live in dry and cold places if the air is clean and fresh. Unnecessary accumulation of water in the surroundings makes the atmosphere humid. Thus drainage of water should be properly regulated. Dirty heaps of waste products are also one of the causes of air pollution. This problem can be solved by burning waste products. But fire produces smoke which is a major pollutant. So this should be done in a place far away from residential areas. At present, vehicular traffic is the main cause of air pollution, particularly in the big cities. To overcome this problem serious efforts are being made the world over.

It is important to keep the atmosphere inside houses clean. Every room should be provided with at least one door and window in addition to ventilators. Freshness of the room environment is inversely proportional to the number of persons in a room. Therefore care should be taken to see that rooms are not overcrowded.

Geographical conditions are responsible for the quality of air. Places at a higher altitude are less polluted as the air is cleaner.

A house with proper ventilation is essential for good health.

Sometimes only a change of climate could cure a patient from an illness.

Food and Drink

Nobody can survive without food and drink which are the primary sources of nutrition for the human body. The quality and quantity of food and drink are important as far as maintaining good health is concerned. Food must be pure and fresh and the diet must be a balanced one. Drinks include water and milk and beverages like tea, coffee and even liquor.

Water. Water is a natural drink and imperative for survival. It helps in absorbing food and makes excretion possible. The quality of water affects the health of a person and quality depends on the source of water. Thus, water that comes from streams and rocky fountains is the best because it contains very little impurity. The next best source is well water. Wells should be deep and covered and the water should constantly be used. In villages, sometimes lakes and ponds are used as sources of water. Pond water is the worst source because water in a pond stagnates and a lot of waste products are found near the pond. Such stagnant and polluted water is the cause of all water-borne diseases. However, if no other source of water is available, this water can be used after boiling or by other methods of purification.

Some principles mentioned by Unani physicians regarding water and health are given below:

1. Drinking plenty of water, particularly during summer is essential for the body.
2. One should avoid drinking water during meals. Drinking water half an hour after a meal is good for digestion.
3. Water which is either too cold or too hot should not be drunk. Lukewarm water is best for the body.
4. Water must be drunk slowly while sitting.

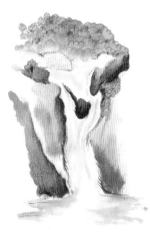

Water from a stream is the purest, rich in minerals and without impurities.

5. It is best to store water in a clay pot as clay keeps the water cool and free from dust particles.

Milk: The first thing a baby drinks is mother's milk: there is no better substitute for this because it not only nourishes the baby but also provides resistance against diseases. To be physically strong from the very beginning, every child should be breast-fed. The mother's health is also important. During lactation, the diet of the mother should be well-balanced.

Even after the infant has been weaned from mother's milk, milk should be an essential part of his or her diet. An individual should try to include either milk or a milk product like yoghurt in his or her diet as long as possible to keep diseases at bay. Milk should always be consumed after boiling.

Beverages: Consumption of beverages vary according to season. Beverages like tea and coffee can become addictive, too much tea or

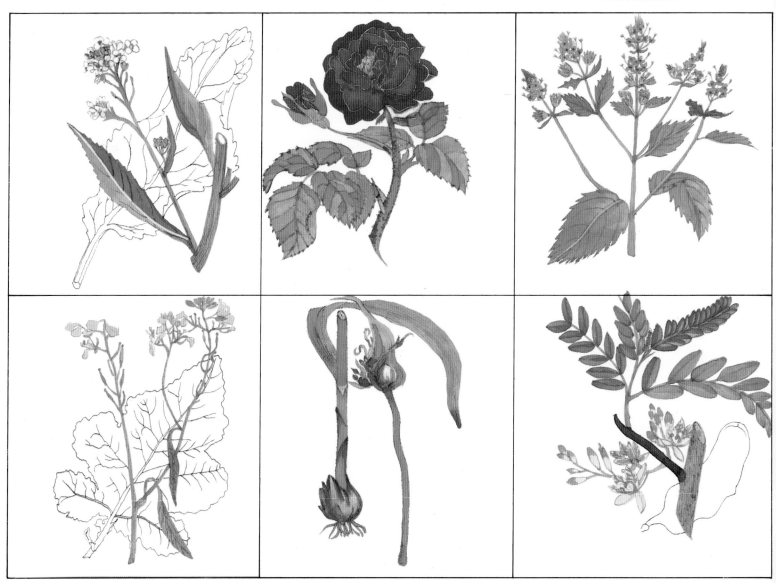

HORSE RADISH

ROSE

PEPPERMINT

BLACK MUSTARD

GARLIC

TAMARIND

All parts of herbs—flowers, roots, leaves, stalks—are used in Unani for medicinal purposes.

coffee is bad for health as that could cause gastritis and constipation. During a typically tropical summer, fruit and vegetable juices help to maintain stamina, most of which is lost due to excessive perspiration. Aerated drinks also help in making up for the water lost from the body. However, these drinks are useful only when they are fresh and pure, otherwise they can harm the body.

Amongst alcoholic beverages, wine and beer help to digest a meal as they help in the absorption of food during the digestive process. They also increase body heat by accelerating the rate of metabolic activities. But excessive drinking of alcohol is harmful for health, especially for the liver. Alcohol also has an adverse effect on the brain and nerves.

Food: It has always been understood that food is the most important requirement of a living being. Food may be defined as anything which nourishes or supplies

Although alcoholic beverages in moderation have their advantages, Unani physicians prohibit them in excess.

building material or energy for the body by strengthening its vital forces. Without eating enough an individual will fall prey to disease and decay. Eating the proper kind of food in the right quantity is imperative for maintaining good health.

It is important to analyse the food that one eats, particularly for its calorific and nutritional value. The concept of a balanced diet was important even to the early Unani physicians.

Principles about Eating

1. Meals should be eaten regularly and on time. It is important to chew the food properly before swallowing.
2. One should not eat so much that one feels heavy and ill. It is important to avoid indigestion as it can lead to other diseases.
3. Food should be cooked properly with moderate amounts of fat and spices.

4. It is important to have a sense of variety in the food one eats.

5. Some rest after lunch and a walk after dinner is very useful. Mental work should not be undertaken immediately after a meal.

Body Movement and Repose

A balance between movement and repose is a must for good health. Movement acts on the body in its own way. If frequency of movement is high and duration is short, then all metabolic activities become faster, leading to excessive heat generation, rapid blood circulation and perspiration. On the other hand, if frequency of movement is low but duration is long, it dissolves the body compounds by utilizing the stored energy which exists in the form of fat.

Repose is just the reverse of movement. It decreases the heat content in the body as the rate and intensity of metabolic activities decrease when the body is in a state of rest. Rest is important as it helps in regaining the energy lost

Ghiza-e-mutadil or a balanced diet.

Mental Movement and Repose

Excessive stimulation of the nerves is harmful for health. Therefore, Unani physicians say there should always be a balance between nervous movement and repose. Nervous excitement leads to several diseases, specially of the heart. Anxiety and mental tension stimulate the nerves which increases the secretion of chemical substances found in the body causing constriction in the blood vessels which in turn leads to hypertension.

Sleeping Habits

During sleep, all activities of the body are suspended, particularly those which are voluntary. As a result, there is not much energy lost. The body also regains lost energy during sleep. Hence after a sound sleep, physical and mental fatigue disappear and the individual feels invigorated. In a day, six to eight hours sleep is essential for a normal adult.

However, excessive sleep makes the body lethargic. Staying awake generates heat in the body owing to the high frequency of metabolic activities and extra calories are burnt away. Thus, a balance between sleep and staying awake is a must to maintain health.

Badam *or almond helps in strengthening powers of immunity.*

Retention and Evacuation

The human body is made of living matter which requires nutrition for the body's functions and growth. Nutrition comes from food. The food passes through various organs and processes till it is assimilated into the body. But all the food is not retained in the body; some waste products are formed during the process of digestion.

Retention of nutritive agents inside the body and excretion of waste products are important for its sustenance. Any alteration or variation in this process can lead to many types of diseases.

Constipation which is a form of natural retention is enough to cause diseases associated with the digestive system. Unnatural excretion like bleeding in excess is sufficient to cause death.

Therefore, it is important to keep an eye on our habits of excretion. We must observe the regularity, quality, quantity, colour and odour of our excretory products. For example, the act of defecation should happen once in every twenty-four hours. The colour of the stool should be dark brown, semi-solid and a quarter of the food eaten.

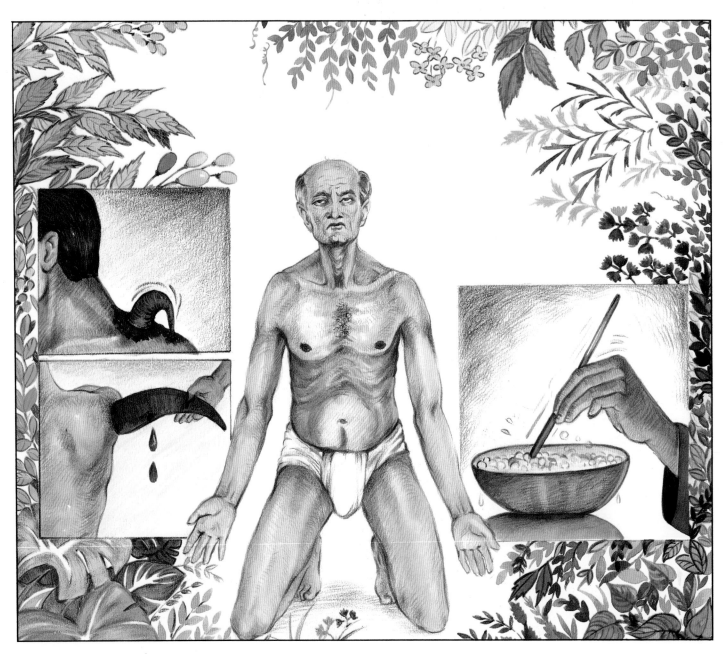

Some typical surgical procedures used in Unani medicine.

Concept Of Diseases
and their Cure

———— ✳ ————

In Unani medicine, the concept of diseases is discussed according to the laws of pathology or *ilmul amraaz* which studies the abnormalities in the structure and function of the body. Broadly, the study is based on three factors: cause or *sabab*, disease or *marz* and after-effect or *arz* .

Cause

Cause or *sabab* can be defined as a specific disturbance which changes the state of the body either from health to sickness or from sickness to health. Here, only those causes are discussed which are responsible in making the body unhealthy, known

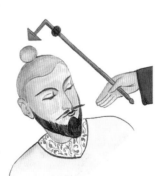

Amal-e-kai *or cauter-ization. An important surgical method.*

as *asbab-e-marz* or causes of diseases.

Causes of diseases can be divided into two types: external causes or *asbab-e-badia* and internal causes or *asbab-e-batina*. External causes are those which affect the body from outside such as excessive hot or cold climate, a polluted atmosphere, injury from an accident etc. Internal causes are those which appear and affect the body internally such as formation of stones inside the kidney or bladder.

Disease

A disease or *marz* is an abnormal condition of the body provoked by a cause. Diseases are classified by Unani physicians in two categories i.e. simple and compound.

Simple disease

Simple diseases are divided into three types on the basis of their causes:

- Abnormal temperament or *sue mizaj*,
- Abnormal structure or *sue tarkeeb*,
- Abnormal dis-continuity and adhesion or *ta farruque wa ittisaal*.

Abnormal temperament: The concept of normal or abnormal temperament in Unani philosophy is based on the theory of humours which has been explained in Chapter 2. Majority of diseases are caused

by an imbalance in the humours. Examples of this kind of disease are diabetes mellitus in which blood sugar level becomes abnormal and hypertension in which blood volume increases.

Abnormal structure: Abnormal structure or malformation of the body is either congenital or acquired. An example is the disease hydrocephalus, a condition in which there is an excessive accumulation of fluid inside the cerebral cavity which affects the structure of the cranial bones.

Abnormal dis-countinuity and adhesion: This category covers all the diseases arising from injuries either surgical or accidental which infect the body and through abnormal healing of wounds and abscesses.

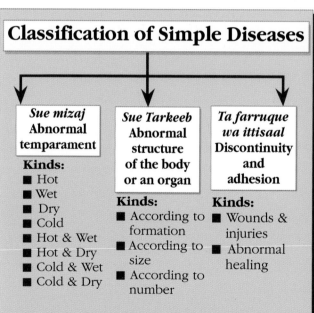

Classification of Simple Diseases

Sue mizaj
Abnormal temparament

Kinds:
- Hot
- Wet
- Dry
- Cold
- Hot & Wet
- Hot & Dry
- Cold & Wet
- Cold & Dry

Sue Tarkeeb
Abnormal structure of the body or an organ

Kinds:
- According to formation
- According to size
- According to number

Ta farruque wa ittisaal
Discontinuity and adhesion

Kinds:
- Wounds & injuries
- Abnormal healing

Compound disease

When two or more simple diseases combine together, it is known as a compound disease. The best example of a compound disease is an abscess which has an abnormal temperament as its components are puss and debris, abnormal structure because of the swelling it causes and abnormal discontinuity because of the tissue damage it brings about.

After-effect

After-effect or *arz* is also an abnormal condition of the body like disease but it happens as a result of a disease. Sometimes, diagnosis of a disease shows a symptom or *alamat.* For example, blood in the urine (hematuria) indicates that there is an injury or a certain type of a pathological condition in the urinary organs or inside the urinary tract.

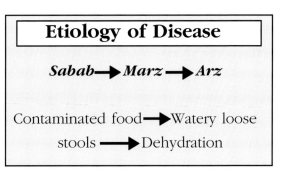

Etiology of Disease

Sabab → *Marz* → *Arz*

Contaminated food → Watery loose stools → Dehydration

Arz is actually the aftermath which follows once the disease has struck which does not determine the exact cause of the disease as an *alamat* can—in diarrhoea, for example, dehydration is a major after-effect. Sometimes, repercussions of one disease cause another disease. If the body breaks into a fever due to an infection, the *arz* which is the fever becomes the disease and causes another *arz* which is bodyache. Thus, a chain forms between *sabab*, *marz* and *arz*.

Ideally, the Unani physician should start his treatment only when he or she has diagnosed the disease after going to the heart of the problem. One cannot rely on the effect of the disease alone. Rehydration may cure dehydration but till it is ensured the food eaten by the patient is free from the risk of infection, the disease will recur.

Find Out Your Temperament

The chart given here helps you understand your temperament. Each temperament is judged according to ten parameters. The reader has to tick on the blank space against the quality which applies to him or her the most amongst all the qualities listed next to each parameter. The next step is to add up all the numbers marked against the qualities chosen and check the total score against the range given below the chart.

	PARAMETER	SANGUINE		PHLEGMATIC		BILIOUS		MELANCHOLIC	
MORPHOLOGICAL	**COMPLEXION**	Ruddy (Reddish/ Wheaty Brown)	1	Chalky (Whitish)	0.75	Pale (Yellowish)	0.5	Purple (Blackish)	0.25
	BUILT	Muscular & Broad	1	Fatty & Broad	0.75	Muscular & Thin	0.5	Skeletal	0.25
	TOUCH	Hot & Soft	1	Cold & Soft	0.75	Hot & Dry	0.5	Cold & Dry	0.25
	HAIR	Black & Lustry Thick, Rapid Growth	1	Black & Thin Slow Growth	0.75	Brown & Thin Rapid Growth	0.5	Brown & Thin Slow Growth	0.25
PHYSIOLOGICAL	**MOVEMENT**	Active	1	Dull	0.75	Hyperactive	0.5	Less Active	0.25
	DIET (MOST LIKED)	Cold & Dry	1	Hot & Dry	0.75	Cold & Moist	0.5	Hot & Moist	0.25
	WEATHER (MOST SUITABLE)	Spring	1	Summer	0.75	Winter	0.5	Autumn	0.25
	SLEEP	Normal (6-8 hours)	1	In excess	0.75	Inadequate	0.5	Insomnia	0.25
	PULSE	Normal in Rate (70-80/ min) Large in Volume	1	Slow in Rate/ (60-70/ min) Normal in Volume	0.75	Rapid in Rate (80/ 100 min) Normal in Volume	0.5	Slow in Rate (60-70/ min) Less in Volume	0.25
PSYCHO-LOGICAL	**EMOTIONS**	Normal	1	Calm & Quiet	0.75	Angry	0.5	Nervous	0.25

SIGNS OF TEMPERAMENT

Total [ ]

Range of Temprament in Numbers:
- Sanguine: 7.51 to 10,
- Phlegmatic: 5.10 to 7.50,
- Bilious: 2.51 to 5.00,
- Melancholic: 0.00 to 2.50

Methods of Diagnosis

Methods of diagnosis are based on the following:

1. General physical examination.
2. Systemic examination.
3. Interrogation.
4. Day-to-day observations.

General Physical Examination

This examination helps determine the patient's temperament. Human temperament is based on the proportion in which the four humours are found in an individual body. There are four types of temperaments found in all human beings as we have already discussed before. Individual temperament can be determined by keeping in mind certain factors like: complexion, built, touch, hair, movements, diet, weather, sleep, pulse rate and emotions.

By observing and assessing these ten parameters, the physician can

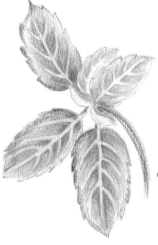

Faranj muskh *or basil. An effective drug for respiratory disorders.*

determine the temperament of a person and the state of the patient's body i.e. whether healthy or unhealthy.

The following inferences could help to indicate the four types of temperaments:

(1) If the complexion is ruddy, the built is muscular, the touch is warm, the hair is thick and shiny, movements are easy, the diet is balanced, the weather which suits the individual's temperament is cold and dry, the individual sleeps enough, the pulse is strong and normal and emotions are controlled and not high-strung, then this type of person has a sanguine temperament or a *damwi mizaj* which is moist and hot by nature.

(2) If the complexion is pale and white, the built is heavy and bulky, the touch is cold and soft, the hair is thin, movements are very little, pulse is slow and diet is reasonably balanced, the weather which is most suitable

for the individual is hot and dry and the individual is not very emotional, then this type of person has a phlegmatic temperament or a *balghami mizaj*.

(3) If the complexion is yellowish, the built is thin, the touch is hot and dry, hair is thin and rough, there is enough movement, the diet is a balanced one, the weather which is most conducive is cold and moist, the pulse is rapid and strong and the person is rather irritable by nature, then this type of person has a bilious temperament or a *safravi mizaj*.

(4) If the complexion is blackish, the frame is frail and weak, the touch is cold and dry, hair is thin and rough but grows quickly, movements are feeble, the diet is neither balanced nor enough, the weather which suits the individual is a warm and moist one, the pulse is slow, then this type of a person has a

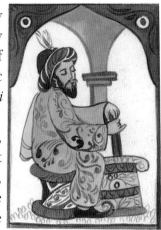

An ancient Unani physician preparing drugs.

melancholic temperament or a *saudavi mizaj*.

Systemic Examination

In the Unani system of medicine, examining and diagnosing a patient for disease is done by determining the state of his faculties. There are mainly three types of faculties in the body which are responsible for performing most body functions. These have been enlisted before. The method of diagnosis in determining the normal or abnormal functioning of these faculties are based on the physical body functions, pulse, urine and stool.

Physical Body Functions: The proper functioning of the physical body is very important for the general well-being of the body as well as the health of a specific organ. The dysfunctioning and malfunctioning of a particular body part would immediately indicate disease and the failure to sustain metabolic activity. The physical body is also very closely related to mental health.

If all the organs in the body perform their activities and are allowed adequate rest, the mental faculty functions perfectly. If otherwise, there is cause for alarm as then this faculty becomes imbalanced.

Pulse: Pulse or *nabz* is a movement based on the expansion and relaxation of the arteries. Three factors are essential to form a pulse which are movements of the heart, arteries and blood. The heart is the source which enables the arteries to move and this movement is conducted through the blood. When the heart contracts, the arteries expand, when the heart relaxes, the arteries contract. Due to the pressure of the blood, arteries expand with every beat or contraction of the heart. The heart then plays an active role to build up blood pressure in the arteries. Thus the heart, blood and the blood vessels are essential to form a pulse. Examining the pulse

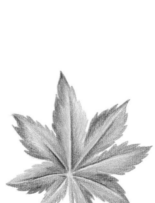

Bedanjeer or castor plant. Applying castor leaves on an abscess helps it mature and heal.

could reveal diseases of the heart and lungs, in other words, dysfunctioning of the *quwat-e-haiwaniya* or the vital faculty of the body.

Urine: Urine or *boul* is a liquid excretory product excreted through the kidneys. The quality and quantity of urine indicates the normal and abnormal states of the body. For determining quality: the colour of the urine, odour, sediments, transparency and viscosity are observed. These factors can change due to climatic conditions, intake of water, type of food eaten and the use of drugs. But some specific changes occur in each of these parameters if there is a disease which help the physician in his diagnosis.

Stool: Stool or *baraz* is a waste product formed as a result of the food which is undigested. It has certain characteristics vis-a-vis colour, odour, volume and consistency which help determine the state of the body. In case of a disease, there could be a change in the character of

45

the stool specially if there is a problem in digestion. Not only the character of stool, the time, duration and frequency of defecation help in diagnosis. At present, the examination and analysis of urine and stool are easy due to the facilities provided by sophisticated laboratories.

Interrogation

After being acquainted with the problem, the physician has to interrogate the patient. This involves questioning the patient about past and present health problems and family history of diseases. In Unani medicinal parlance, the process of interrogation is known as *sariryat*.

Day-to-day Observations

In the Unani system of medicine, the pathology of a disease is classified in various stages i.e. the beginning or *ibtida*, acceleration or *tazaiyud*, saturation or *intaba* and retardation

Tablets are coated with silver to protect them from climatic influences.

or *inhetat* . Hence, in each stage, the disease requires a different type of treatment. Therefore, a daily observation of the patient is essential. It is essential for the physician to first diagnose the stage of the disease. Ultimately it is in the hands of nature, which gives the body the power of *tabiat*, to supervise the process of healing after the disease has passed through the four stages. For example, an abscess which causes white puss to form reaches its peak, ruptures and then heals. During its many stages, the abscess requires different kinds of treatment. In the first stage, the doctor has to prescribe medicines which will mature it; next the medicine has to assist rupturing and finally heal the wound.

Laws of Treatment

In the Unani system of medicine, the laws of treatment are based on the

46

theory of temperament, particularly on the concept and functions of the normal and homeostatic temperament. This concept states that all the elements of a compound have to be perfectly balanced according to their quantity and quality to be able to perform the required functions. The body is also a compound of various types of matter. Matter is divided broadly into three physical states i.e. solid, liquid and gaseous. A physician has to try to maintain the normal temperament of an individual which is equivalent to maintaining the normal quantity and quality of the body humours.

The quality of the humours are based on four basic qualities i.e. hot, cold, dry and wet. The combination of either two of these qualities forms the temperament of each. Thus their temperaments can be hot and wet, hot and dry, cold and wet and cold and dry. Every organ of the body also has its own temperament. The heart is said to be hot and wet, liver; hot and dry, the brain is cold and

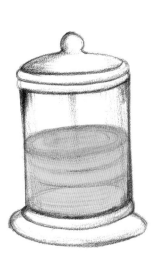

Massage with oil helps to avoid friction and invigorates the skin.

wet and the spleen is cold and dry in nature. Thus, a physician has to aim at maintaining the normal temperament of each organ as well as the whole body of a patient.

In Unani medicine, if the disease is of a particular temperament, the drug prescribed is usually of the opposite one so that it can neutralise the effect of the disease. A disease which is hot in nature can be cured by a drug which is temperamentally cold.

Lines of Treatment

The Unani physician follows four methods of treatment: regimental therapy, diet-o-therapy, pharmaco-therapy and surgery. Out of these four, the physician likes to use that line of treatment which is closest to nature. Regimental therapy is usually preferred because it eliminates the risks of harming the body. If regimental therapy fails in curing the disease, other methods are used.

For example, if a person is obese, the physician advises him first to exercise. Excessive rest causes accumulation of fat inside the body. By exercising, heat is generated which dissolves the fat. But, if exercise fails, the physician has to reduce or alter the diet of the patient. If this too does not solve the problem, the physician can use pharmacotherapy: with the help of some natural drugs try to dissolve excess fat in the body. This type of weight-reducing drugs are known as *muhazzil*. If all these methods of treatment fail to reduce obesity, then the physician has to resort to surgery, which is considered the most unnatural form of treatment as it may harm the body in many ways.

Modes of Regimental Therapy

1. EXERCISE: Exercise or *riyazat* may be defined as a voluntary and rhythmic movement an individual makes with one or more parts of the body to expend excess energy. It

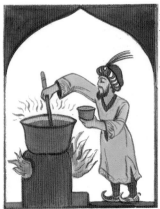

A typical Unani pharmaceutical method to extract oil from a herb.

is usually accompanied by breathlessness.

Purpose:

- It hardens the organs and renders them fit to perform their functions.
- It results in better absorption of food, aids assimilation, increases innate heat of the body and improves nutrition.
- It clears the pores of the skin.
- It removes waste products through the lungs.
- It strengthens the physique.

2. MASSAGE: Massage or *dalak* may be defined as rubbing and kneading a part of the body with the fingers or palm of the hand or other objects like a rough cloth.

Varieties of friction:
- Hard friction
- Moderately hard friction
- Rough friction
- Soft or gentle friction

Purpose:
- Hard friction stretches, contracts and braces the body.

48

- Soft friction has a relaxing effect.
- Repeated friction reduces body fat.
- Rough friction which is done with a rough towel draws the blood rapidly to the surface and enhances circulation.
- Gentle friction is massage with moderate force. It is usually done by using the palm or a soft towel. It increases and maintains the blood circulation of an organ.

3. STEAM BATH: In a steam bath or *hammam*, the body is immersed in hot water or steam.

Purpose:
- It releases waste products and impurities through the skin.
- It reduces the viscosity of the humours of the body
- It reduces obesity.

4. FOMENTATION: Fomentation or *takmeed* is the process of keeping the body or a part of the body warm with the help of a piece of cloth which is hot. The heat should not

Hammam or steam bath is part of the therapy.

exceed the tolerance level of the patient.

Purpose:
- To get relief from pain.
- To help subside swelling in a particular area of the body.

5. EMESIS: Emesis or vomiting or *qae* involves the excretion of gastric contents through the mouth.

Purpose:
- The main purpose of the act is to eliminate toxic substances from the stomach.

6. PURGING: Purging or *ishaal* involves the excretion of waste matter through the bowels.

Purpose:
- This too is an attempt to free the body of toxic substances.

7. ENEMA: Enema or *huqnah* is a method in which liquids are introduced into the rectum by an object through the anal canal.

Purpose:
- To get rid of the superfluities in the intestinal tract.
- To reduce pain in the bladder and kidneys
- To relieve inflammatory conditions in the organs surrounding the rectum
- To relieve colic pain.

Note: *All methods of regimental therapy mentioned should be followed in consultation with a physician.*

Diet-o-Therapy

The aim of diet-o-therapy or *ilaj-bil-ghiza* is to treat ailments by regulating the quality and quantity of the patient's diet. The most important aspect of this treatment is to alter the quality of food as far as ingredients and physical state are concerned.

Prohibition of food or *tark-e-ghiza* is prescribed when the physician wants to give complete rest to the patient's digestive system

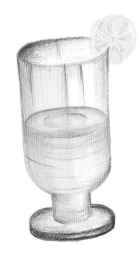

Ghiza-e-lateef *or liquid diet, advised in cases of digestive failure.*

in a very advanced stage of a disease.

Restriction of food or *taqleel-e-ghiza* is prescribed when the physician wants to give rest to the digestive system yet at the same time wants the patient to regain strength through certain nutritive foods. Such a therapy is advised in cases of obesity, diabetes etc.

Eating excess food or *ifrat-e-ghiza* is suggested when the patient is undernourished or malnourished. It is also suggested if the requirement of the body is more than normal, for eg. an athlete would require more food than an ordinary person with sedentary habits.

Alteration in diet or *tabdeel-e-ghiza* is suggested when the patient's body condition requires a change in diet. The following are some examples of this kind of treatment:

Liquid diet: A liquid diet or *ghiza-e-lateef* is given in the case of a digestive failure. Fruit juices, soups of different vegetables, mutton and chicken may be taken.

Semi-solid diet: A semi-solid diet or *ghiza-e-mutawassat* is prescribed in the case of poor digestion. A light diet comprising curds *or khichri* (gruel) is recommended when the patient is unable to digest normal food.

Normal diet: A normal diet or *ghiza-e-mutadil* could be given to a healthy individual to maintain good health and sustain body strength to fight diseases. An ideal diet should be balanced and sufficient in carbohydrates proteins, fats, vitamins and minerals.

Pharmacotherapy

In pharmacotherapy or *ilaj-bid-dawa,* drugs are prescribed which are in their most natural form derived from natural sources i.e. herbal, mineral and animal. Herbal drugs, however, dominate this system. As the drugs are natural in form, they suit the body and have very little side-effects. If a drug contains toxic properties in its crude

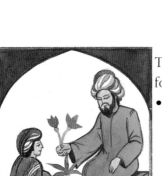
Herbal drugs dominate in the Unani system.

form, it is purified before administering.

The Greek and Arab physicians encouraged polypharmacy and devised a large number of polypharmaceutical recipes which are still in use. In the Unani system, although medicines composed of a single drug are preferred, a compound formulation of drugs is also prescribed in the treatment of various complex and chronic diseases.

Rules of Drug Administration

There are a few basic rules to be followed in selecting medicines.

- *Selection according to quality:* It is important to select drugs on the basis of temperament i.e. whether the drug is hot, cold, moist or dry.
- *Selection in terms of amount prescribed:* There are two sub-divisions in this case : measurement in terms of weight and measurement based on the

degree of intensity of the drug's effect.

The drugs which act very fast are referred to as poison or *sum* because they change the internal environment of the body very swiftly. Sometimes, the patient is unable to tolerate this sudden change and dies. So physicians use these drugs in particularly unavoidable circumstances with a great deal of caution. The knowledge of drugs and their dosage is very important because the Unani physician believes that every drug has the potential to become poisonous if not taken in the right dosage and can cure only when the appropriate amount is administered.

Besides those mentioned above, there are other factors which determine dosage such as the physician's knowledge of the malady, the nature of the organs affected, the degree of intensity of the illness, the patient's age, lifestyle, geographical location, occupation, strength and physique.

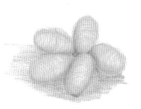
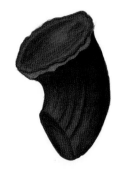
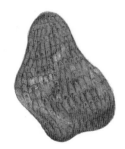

Some widely-used drugs of animal origin.

Single drug therapy: In single drug therapy, either one or more than one drug may be prescribed, but all the drugs should be in their crude single form and not be combined in the form of a compound.

Compound drug therapy: In compound drug therapy, a compound consisting of two or more drugs may be prescribed.

Surgery

Surgery or *jarahat* should be resorted to when all other ways have failed and there is a need for extreme measures. The ancient physicians of Unani medicine were pioneers in the field of surgery and developed their own instruments and techniques. But at present only minor forms of surgery are practised in this system. They are as follows:

1. VENESECTION: Venesection or *fasd* is a surgical process in which a blood vessel, a vein in particular is cut open by a surgical knife to shed excessive or impure blood.

Purpose:
- When there is so much excessive or unhealthy blood that a disease is about to develop, venesection is a preventive procedure.
- When a disease is already present, venesection can be a curative measure.

2. CUPPING: Cupping or *hijamat* is a method of local evacuation. It removes excess quantity of humours accumulated in a part of the body or helps in collecting the humours in a localised area of the body by a method in which first vacuum is created in a cup-like container which is then placed over a certain part of the body.

Purpose:
- The operation of cupping cleanses the body, specially when there is a subdermal accumulation of waste products or fluids.

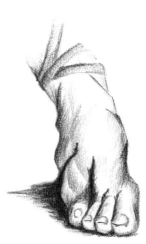

Fasd *or venesection. A method of surgery used to shed impure blood.*

- It helps to release the rarefied rather than the more viscous blood from the body.

3. LEECHING: Leeching or *taleeque* is an ancient method of local evacuation through the use of leeches.

Purpose:
- To remove impure or infected blood from the body, particularly when the impure blood has gone deep inside the body.

4. CAUTERIZATION: Cauterization or *amal-e-kai* is a method of treatment in which direct heat or a corrosive agent is applied to the body.

Purpose:
- To coagulate blood.
- To remove unhealthy flesh.
- To remove infection.
- To strengthen the weak parts of the body.
- To act as a stimulant.
- To prevent the spread of a destructive lesion like a septic wound.

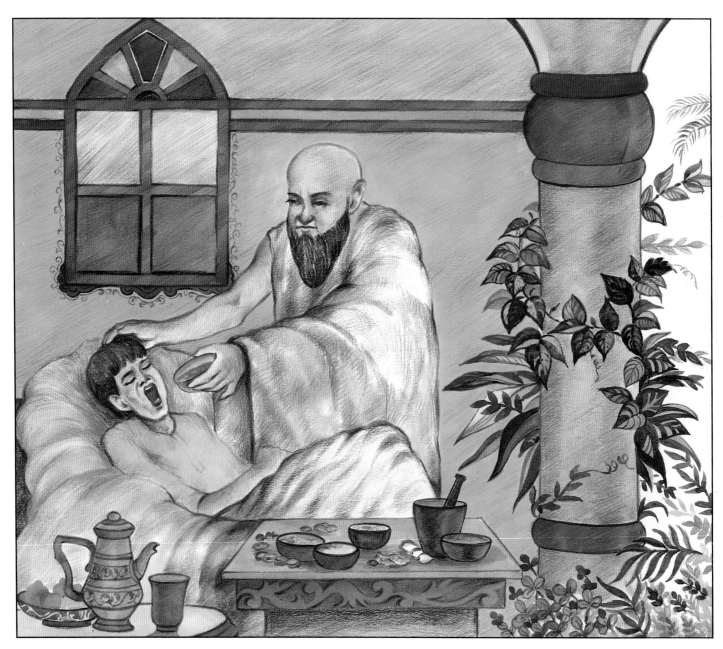

A Unáni physician tending to a patient. The patient is kept close to nature during illness.

Home Remedies

——— ✳ ———

The Unani system of medicine offers remedies for many diseases. This chapter deals only with those diseases which are common and non-fatal. Readers can follow these remedies at home without consulting a physician. If these remedies are not effective or cause other complications, it is best to consult a physician.

COMMON FEVER
(Humma-e-umoomi)

Except in cases where there are other complications or where the exact cause of the fever is unknown or the temperature goes too far beyond the normal range, no medication is necessary because such a fever might be nature's way of getting rid of the

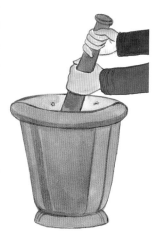

A type of grinder (kharal) used in preparing Unani medicines.

various poisons accumulated in the body.

Treatment

If the fever does not subside or if it goes far beyond the normal limit, the first thing to do is to wash the forehead of the patient with cold water in which rose water and a little vinegar has been mixed. Cold compresses should be kept on the head if the temperature is above 103° F. If inspite of the cold compress the fever continues to rise and reaches 106° F, emergency procedures should be started immediately. The clothes of the patient should be removed and he or she should be wrapped in a cotton sheet dipped in ice-cold water with a blanket wrapped over the sheet. The temperature will then start coming down. The sheet should be changed every fifteen minutes.

Or the patient can be bathed in cold water. When the temperature comes down to 103° F, only a cold compress on the head will do. At the first signs of temperature falling, cold compresses should also be discontinued.

During fever, the patient should not eat. The only thing that a patient suffering from fever should be allowed is fruit juice. Juice of lemon in a glass of water with a pinch of salt is very useful. The patient must also drink plenty of water . Lack of liquids may lead to dehydration which is much more difficult to cure than ordinary fever.

CONSTIPATION (*Husra*)

When the waste matter is not released from the intestines, it is known as constipation. Lack of exercise and consumption of rich food leads to putrefaction and

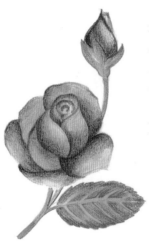

Gule-e-surkh *or rose. Confection of rose petals is used as a laxative.*

formation of flatus in the stomach; sometimes the whole abdomen is distended causing acute discomfort.

Remedies

1. The best way to deal with constipation is to change food habits. Milk, boiled vegetables, fruits and their juices should be taken in large quantities together with foods containing a lot of rough and fibrous matter.

2. Ten grams of senna (*Cassia angustifolia*) and five grams of aniseed should be boiled in a cup of water with jaggery (*gur*), an extract of *Saccharum officinarum*, then strained and drunk before retiring for the night.

3. Half a litre of milk mixed with 50 gm of brown sugar (*khand*) taken at night will give relief.

4. Another remedy is to eat 40 gm of Gulkand (*Rosa damascena*), a confection of rose petals, with milk everyday.

5. If these remedies fail to give relief, six grams of the rind of *harad* (*Terminalia chebula*) should be finely ground and mixed with a little salt and lukewarm water and then drunk.

DYSPEPSIA (*Tukhma*)

A weak digestive system coupled with overeating or eating heavy, spicy foods leads to dyspepsia. Delayed digestion of such foods leads to putrefaction of the matter in the stomach and the intestines. There is a feeling of an extremely full stomach, loss of appetite and general discomfort. The patient may feel nausea as well. Belching would leave a sour taste in the mouth.

Remedies

In the case of nausea, it is better to induce vomiting by taking lukewarm water to which a teaspoonful of salt has been added. After the patient has vomited, he should be given 3 gm of white cumin seeds and 1 gm of salt with 10 ml of vinegar. If nausea still

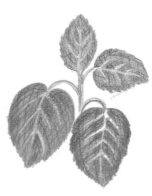

Nana or mint is used chiefly for digestive problems.

persists, 6 gm of mint leaves boiled in water to which 3 gm of small cardamom has been added could be given to the patient to drink.

DIARRHOEA (*Ishaal*)

Diarrhoea may occur in an individual due to many reasons: harmful bacteria during cholera, dietary indiscretions in typhoid fever, ulceration of the intestines in tuberculosis or some diseases of the liver or pancreas.

Remedies

1. The first measure to take in diarrhoea is to begin a diet entirely comprising liquids. One must drink plenty of water because lack of water may lead to dehydration.
2. If diarrhoea occurs due to weak intestines, pills made of *amla* (*Emblica officinalis*) soaked in water to which a pinch of salt has been added may be given to the patient daily in the morning and evening.

3. If the kernel of an old mango is available, it may be roasted with an equal quantity of powdered aniseed. This may be taken in six-gram doses in the morning and evening.
4. Ten grams of *doodhi* (*Euphorbia hirta*) ground in water could be drunk to check diarrhoea, or a paste made of the inner bark of the mango tree may be applied around the navel.
5. Fresh pulp of bael fruit *(Aegle marmelos)* roasted and taken in twenty-gram doses also helps stop diarrhoea.

Regimen

Lime juice added to water with a pinch of salt is the best drink during diarrhoea as it prevents dehydration.

FLATULENCE *(Nafakh)*

Formation of gas or flatus in the stomach is primarily due to improper digestion. Waste matter goes on putrefying in the intestines and leads

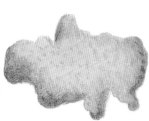

Heeng *or asafoetida, used to treat flatulence.*

to severe flatulence and distension of the stomach.

Remedies

1. A piece of cloth or cotton wool soaked in hot water which has asafoetida (*heeng*) dissolved in it may be used for fomenting the abdomen.
2. Six grams of turpentine oil may be mixed with double the quantity of castor oil and applied on the abdomen. Also, warm leaves of the castor tree may be wrapped over the abdomen.

DYSENTERY (*Zaheer*)

Dysentery is a condition in which there is an inflammation of the lower intestines, colic pain in the region of the abdomen and liquid or semi-formed stools with mucus and blood. It may be caused by certain organisms but in many cases it is the result of dietary indiscretions like eating very spicy foods, fried and hard-to-digest-fatty substances. The patient is severely constipated. There may even be a burning sensation at the time of passing stool. If there is blood in the stools, it indicates the bacillary type of dysentery. The other kind is the amoebic dysentery.

Remedies

1. Of all the home remedies, the bael fruit is perhaps the most effective in the treatment of dysentery of both varieties. The pulp of this fruit should be taken a few times during the day.
2. Ten grams of *kurchi (Holerrhena antidysenterica)* bark, the pulp of the bael fruit, poppy seeds and white cumin should be finely ground and four grams of this powder may be taken with water.

Regimen

The first thing to do in the case of dysentery is to stop all hard-to-digest, spicy, fatty foods. The patient should be kept on a diet of thin gruel made of split green gram *(Phaseolus mungo)* and rice. Or he may be given soup and bread without any butter.

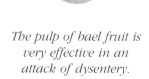

The pulp of bael fruit is very effective in an attack of dysentery.

INTESTINAL PARASITES
(*Kirm-e-Shikam*)

The most common parasites which infest the human intestines are: round worms, tape worms, hook worms, thread worms and giardia. The presence of these worms in the intestines causes a voracious appetite, diarrhoea, anaemia and headache. The presence of worms in stool should never be neglected: their continued presence may lead to obstruction in the intestines and the bile duct, giving rise to further complications.

Remedies

1. The treatment of this illness lies primarily in the patient's diet. The patient' meals should be light, non-spicy, fatless, easily digestible and bland.
2. *Bahera (Terminalia belerica)* and the seeds of *palash (Butea frondosa)* are the best medicines to counter this disease. One teaspoonful of

these herbs daily would be very effective.

3. In case of tape worm, boil the bark of a pomegranate tree in half a litre of water till a quarter of the water is left. Divide this mixture into three equal doses and take them in regular one-hour intervals. After the last dose, it is advisable to take 40 gm of castor oil.

CONJUNCTIVITIS (*Ramad*)

This is a disorder of the eyes. In this malady the affected eye becomes red or bloodshot. There is a feeling of sand having entered the eye and also pain in some cases.

Remedies

1. The first step in the treatment of conjunctivitis is to keep the eyes clean; they should be washed with hot water in which a little borax has been dissolved.

2. A concoction made of candied sugar, alum and rock salt (3 gm

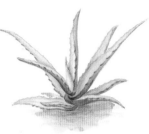

Gheekawar *or the aloe plant helps in combating conjunctivitis.*

each), 6 gm of *rasaut (Berberis aristata)* and 117 ml of rose water should be used as an eye drop.

3. A paste made of aloe (*Aloe barbadensis*), large *harad*, and alum (4 gm each), 1 gm of opium ground together in a little water should be applied over the eyelids.

STYE (*Shaeirah*)

This begins as a general swelling of the eyelid accompanied by pain, which gradually suppurates. The inflammation is restricted to the sebaceous glands.

Remedies

1. One of the best remedies for styes is clove. A clove ground and mixed with water should be applied over the stye.

2. Applying the paste of a date kernel ground in water also has a medicinal effect in this condition.

ODONTITIS
(Jiryan-ud-dum-lissah)

Odontitis is a condition in which the teeth bleed and become loose. It precedes or is a concomitant of pyorrhoea and must be dealt with by maintaining oral hygiene and the following remedies.

Remedies

1. A fine powder of 20 gm of oak gall or *muzu* (*Quercus infectoria*) and 6 gm of alum should be used as tooth powder. The teeth and the gums should be vigorously rubbed with it and the mouth washed after half an hour of applying to allow the powder to have its full effect.
2. If the fresh bark of acacia or *babul* tree is chewed daily, loose teeth will become firm and the gums will stop bleeding.
3. A decoction of 20 gm of the bark of *moolsari* (*Mimusops elengi*) boiled in half a litre of water till about 250 ml is left should be used as a mouth wash.

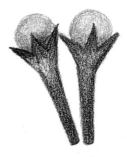

Quaranful *or clove.*
Clove oil relieves toothache.

TOOTHACHE *(Wajaul-asnaan)*

A tooth whose nerve has been exposed by a cavity can be excruciatingly painful. If the nerve is affected, not much can be done as even a pain-killer will only have a temporary effect. The following remedies can be used to deal with an aching tooth.

Remedies

1. A paste made of finely ground leaves of basil or *tulsi (Ocimum sanctum)* should be warmed a little and applied to the aching tooth.
2. Ginger ground into a paste with a pinch of salt also relieves toothache.
3. One decigram of salmiac should be wrapped in a little cottonwool and pressed on the aching tooth. The fluid secreted should be allowed to run out of the mouth.
4. *Baoberang (Embelia ribes)* may be finely powdered and tied in fine muslin bags. These then

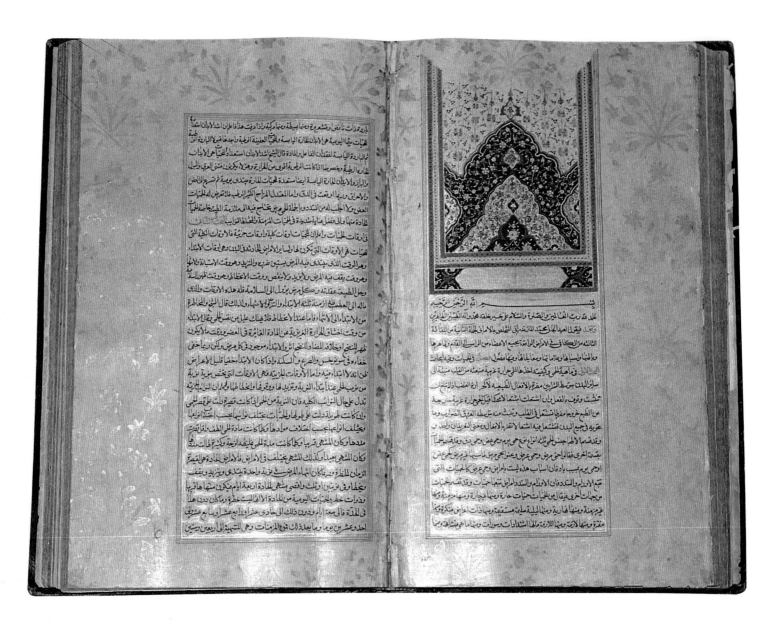

An ancient manuscript of Unani medicine: Kitab-ul-Kafi *(AD 1642).*

should be slightly moistened with water, warmed and applied to the aching tooth to alleviate pain.

5. If the gums are swollen and there is a pervading ache in the whole of the dental structure, 20 gm of dry tobacco leaves and three grams of pepper should be ground together and rubbed on the gums.

6. Applying clove oil is an effective cure.

PREMATURE GREYING
(Shaeb-e-shaar)

Lack of care for the hair, a tendency to wash them with hot water or to dry them with electric dryers are some of the factors which cause hair to grey. Using hair dyes when hair has just started to grey also accelerates the process of greying.

Remedies

1. A vigorous massage of the scalp regularly after washing the hair with cold water should be made a habit.

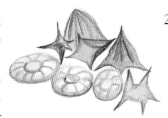

Gokhroo *or small caltrops. A herb used primarily to prevent premature greying.*

2. As for internal remedies, the best is one teaspoonful of moon creeper or *giloya (Tinospora cordiofolia)* and small caltrops or *gokhroo (Tribulus terrestris)* in equal parts mixed with honey taken thrice a day.

3. *Mandur (Erythrina stricta), amla* and *jalapa (Ipomoea purga)* flowers in equal quantities should be ground into a paste and this should be applied to the hair. After the paste dries, the hair should be washed in water in which *amla* has been soaked overnight.

BALDNESS (*Saafah*)

The factors leading to baldness are almost the same as those which contribute to premature greying of hair. Premature baldness is generally hereditary and not much can be done to cure it. If action can be taken when hair starts falling, baldness can be delayed by some months or even years.

Remedies

1. Rubbing oil in which mangoes have been preserved for one year on the scalp helps in pre-empting baldness.

2. If signs of baldness have already appeared, 50 gm of the leaves of *tamarish (Tamarix articulata)* should be ground and made into pellets. These should then be boiled in mustard oil. This oil should be decanted and used for massaging on the bald patches.

PATCHY BALDNESS
(Tanasur-wa-tamrat)

Patchy baldness or alpecia is common on the scalp, but may affect hair all over the body. It occurs mostly among adolescents and young adults.

Remedies

1. Two or three cloves of garlic should be ground together with a pinch of collyrium (a soothing ointment for the eyes) and applied to the hairless patch; if there is any irritation, butter should be smeared over the patch.

2. The bald patch can also be washed with the juice of *amla* and cut with a razor so that a little blood flows out.

ECZEMA *(Nar-e-faarsi)*

Eczema in its acute form shows itself by redness and inflammation of the skin, formation of minute vesicles, and causes severe heat and irritation. If the vesicles rupture, a raw, moist surface is formed from which a colourless liquid is discharged. Eczema may be dry (with only a patch of thick, itchy skin) or weeping, in which there is secretion.

Remedies

1. Twenty grams each of the bark of mango and acacia trees should be boiled in about one litre of water and used to steam the affected part. After this fomentation, the affected part should be smeared with *ghee* (clarified butter).

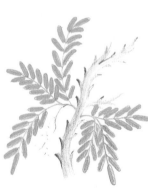

Aqaqia *or the acacia tree. A widely-used medicinal plant, specially effective in eczema.*

2. *Babchi (Psoralea corylifolia)* should be powdered, mixed with mustard oil and applied like an ointment.

3. The leaves of the Indian butter tree or *mahua (Madhuca indica)* should be smeared with sesame oil, warmed over a fire and bandaged on the affected parts. The bandages should be changed every three to four hours.

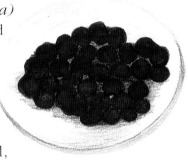

Babchi *or psoralia. Its seeds help in treating leucoderma.*

LEUCODERMA *(Bars)*

In this there is a localised loss of pigmentation of the skin and white patches form on different parts of the body. Although the disease is not fatal, it mars an individual's looks and can be psychologically very disturbing.

Remedies

1. The seeds of *babchi* are particularly useful in leucoderma. The seeds should be soaked in the juice of ginger for three days; the fluid must be replaced after every twenty-four hours. They should then be dried in the shade and ground after their husks have been removed. One gram of this powder should be taken every day with fresh milk for forty days continuously. It could also be applied to the white spots.

2. Equal quantities of *babchi* and tamarind seeds should be soaked in water for three to four days, shelled and dried in the shade. These should be ground and applied to the white patches on the skin for a week. If the paste causes itching, it should be discontinued. When the white spots become red and a fluid is discharged from them, the application should be stopped. If the patches do not burn or itch, *babchi* seeds should be taken internally for forty days.

BOILS AND PUSTULES
(Dumbul & nifaat)

Boils are small areas of inflammation which begin from the root of the

65

hair and are caused by certain infections. The basic cause is bacterial, but many circumstances contribute to the growth of bacteria. If boils are not treated, supplementary boils form around the main growth and cause more pain.

Remedies

1. A leaf of the *peepal* (*Ficus religiosa*) tree smeared with lukewarm clarified butter should be wrapped over the boil. If puss has started to form, it will burst and if it is in its preliminary stages, the growth will subside.
2. An internal remedy for boils and pustules is to grind *brahmadandi* (*Lamprachaenium microcephalum*), mix it in water and add seven grains of pepper. The resultant mixture should be drunk after straining.

PRICKLY HEAT (*Hasaf*)

During the hot summer months and the humid rainy season when the

Gil-e-multani *or marl. A type of soil effective in skin diseases like prickly heat.*

body perspires profusely, small red pustules appear on the body, especially on the chest, back and abdomen. These are the manifestations of what is known as prickly heat.

Remedies

1. Bole Armeniac (*multani mitti*) should be dissolved in water and the thin paste so obtained should be smeared over the affected parts. When the paste has dried, one should scrub oneself with cold water.
2. Green *heena* (*Lawsonia alba*) leaves ground in water can be applied to the affected parts of the skin.

URTICARIA (*Shara*)

Nettle rash or urticaria is a disorder of the skin in which rashes appear all over the body.

Remedies

An easy remedy to prevent repeated

attacks of urticaria is to grind six grams of *jalneem* (*Lycopus europaeus*) and mix it with ten grams of beeswax. This mixture should be dried and made into small round pills. Two such pills could be taken daily with lukewarm water.

NOSE BLEED (*Ruaaf*)

A bleeding nose is not an uncommon condition. There is nothing to worry about if the body heats up because of extreme weather conditions, but if the nose bleeds because of hypertension, there is cause for concern. If it continues for too long and the loss of blood is profuse, only surgical interference may help as copious discharge of blood may indicate the bursting of an artery.

Remedies

1. A person bleeding from the nose should lie on a bed in a position in which the head is higher than the rest of his body. He or she

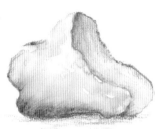

Shibb-e-yamani or alum, a mineral drug which helps to stem bleeding.

should inhale ice-cold water; cold water should be poured over the head and cold compresses applied to the nasal region.

2. Equal quantities of alum, camphor and *majuphala* (*Quercus infectorious*) should be powdered and then inhaled in small doses through the bleeding nose.

3. Applying one decigram of camphor dissolved in the juice of green coriander leaves to the nostrils stops the bleeding fast.

INFLUENZA (*Nazla-e-wabaiyah*)

Influenza generally strikes during the changes of season. Its main symptoms are: irritation and later inflammation of the nose, pharynx and larynx; nose bleed; a dry hacking cough; fever which ranges between 101°F to 102°F and a general bodyache.

Remedies

1. The best remedy for influenza is

perhaps long pepper (*Piper longum*). Half a teaspoon of the powder of long pepper mixed with two teaspoonfuls of honey and half a teaspoonful of the juice of ginger taken thrice daily would nip influenza in the bud if taken in the preliminary stages of the disease.

2. A gram of basil leaves and an equal quantity of dry ginger should be boiled together and drunk as a beverage.

3. Another effective remedy is to drink milk in which a teaspoonful of turmeric powder has been added, thrice a day. This pre-empts the after-effects of influenza and also activates the liver which becomes sluggish during the attack.

COUGH (*Suaal*)

Cough is a condition in which there is irritation in the throat due to an infection and a dry hacking sound is produced as the human system tries to deal with the irritation. It may occur due to inflammation of the larynx or the pharynx.

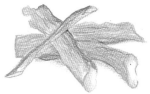

Asl-us-soos or liquorice. This herb is very effective in respiratory disorders; chewing it relieves cough.

Remedies

1. In coughs where there is no phlegm, the throat should be lubricated with a decoction of liquorice or *mulethi (Glycyrrhiza glabra)* root with sugar or honey.

2. A paste made of equal quantities of black raisins, dates, black pepper, *bahera (Terminalia bellirica)*, long pepper and honey could be licked slowly to get quick relief.

3. Ten grams of linseed crushed and boiled in a quarter litre of water (the decoction is ready when half the water is left) taken with 20 gm of honey is a wonderful expectorant.

4. A decoction of *vasaka (Adhatoda vasica)* flowers (50 gm of flowers and thrice their weight of jaggery) eaten in ten-gram doses twice daily relieves cough and even reduces the virulence of pulmonary tuberculosis.

WHOOPING COUGH (Shahiquah)

This is an infectious disease in which at the end of a coughing fit, the patient ends up vomiting which is accompanied by phlegm. The act of vomiting provides temporary relief but the ailment returns unless treated properly.

The disease, fortunately, is not fatal even if it continues for many months.

Remedies

The best home remedy is to take a teaspoonful of ginger juice with an equal quantity of honey twice or thrice a day.

HICCUP (Fovaque)

Hiccups are caused usually by an irritation of the nerves which reaches the diaphragm, making it contract suddenly. They are generally caused by digestive disorders but can also sometimes be a symptom of a serious illness. In extreme cases an attack of hiccups could even signal impending death.

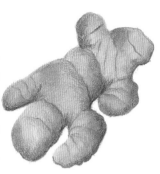

Zanjabeel *or ginger. Ginger juice helps in subsiding cough.*

Remedies

1. Five grams of the ash of peacock feather six times a day with honey is an effective cure for this condition.
2. Another remedy is to keep 20 gm each of warm *ajwain* (*Trachyspermum ammi*) and salt tied in a cloth on the abdomen of the patient.

BRONCHITIS AND BRONCHIAL ASTHMA (Warm-e-shob)

If the tubes which carry air to the lungs become inflamed, the condition is known as bronchitis. Viscous phlegm sticks to the tubes and the air passage is narrowed, resulting in difficulty in breathing. A fit of coughing turns the patient blue and the lack of oxygen leads to progressive weakening.

Remedies

1. The simplest remedy is to take one teaspoonful of turmeric powder (*haldi*) in milk, twice or thrice a day. It should be taken

preferably on an empty stomach.

2. An alternate remedy is a powder made of equal quantities of dried ginger, pepper and long pepper taken thrice daily. This may be mixed with honey or added to a cup of tea.

ASTHMA *(Zeequn-nafas)*

Asthma is a condition in which the passage through which air goes to the lungs becomes narrow leading to difficulty in breathing. This condition may last for a few hours or may linger for some days. If it becomes chronic, the patient acquires the typical asthmatic look, a pale face and an emaciated body.

Remedies and Regimen

Medicines prescribed for cough are also beneficial for asthma in its preliminary stages. If the condition persists for some time expert medical aid should be sought. A walk in the morning is advisable; no other exercise can be encouraged.

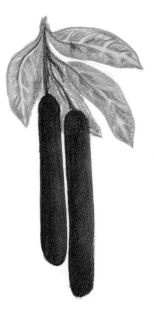

Khayar shambar *or stick plant. The pulp of its fruit is very effective in treating tonsillitis.*

TONSILLITIS *(Warm-e-lauzatain)*

When the tonsils become inflammed, the condition is known as tonsillitis. There is difficulty in swallowing and the patient is unable to eat. Sometimes the glands under the jaws are also inflamed and tender to touch and the pain travels up to the ear.

Remedies

1. The treatment of tonsillitis must start with hot fomentation of the front of the neck.
2. Ten grams of *banafsha* (*Viola odorata*) flowers should be boiled in five times the milk (50 ml), strained and taken hot before going to bed.
3. The bark of acacia (*babul*) should be boiled in water and the decoction used for gargles.
4. Liquorice, *vacha* (*Acorus calamus*) and *kulanjan* (*Alpinia galanga*) should be powdered and mixed with honey. This should be used as a cough expectorant.

Regimen

All hot spicy foods, particularly those in which chillies have been used as an ingredient, must be avoided; bland, soft and liquid foods are the best. Sour substances, curds, buttermilk and fried food too should be shunned.

HOARSENESS *(Bahut-e-saut)*

Inflammation of the throat (particularly the larynx) or even a bad case of tonsillitis may lead to hoarseness of the voice. It may also be precipitated by overusing the larynx or by talking loudly over a long period of time.

Remedies and Regimen

The first thing to do when suffering from a sore throat is to give up all irritating substances like chillies, condiments, sour substances and smoking. The next step is to take saline gargles or gargles with a decoction of acacia bark as advised for tonsillitis. In the case of overuse

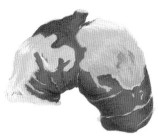

Kulanjan *or Siamese ginger. Chewing its root is the best remedy for a hoarse voice.*

of the vocal chords, *kulanjan* is perhaps the best remedy.

INSOMNIA *(Sahar)*

Sleeplessness or insomnia is a condition in which a person is sluggish and lethargic during the day because he fails to get his natural sleep in the night. Insomnia usually occurs because of stress and anxiety. Hence, its treatment depends on correct diagnosis and subsequent removal of the cause of stress.

Remedies:

1. *Brahmi booti (Herpestis monniera)*, *vacha* and *amla* are the most effective drugs for insomnia. Powders of these drugs, individually or in combination, in doses of one teaspoonful thrice daily with water or milk is the best.
2. A teaspoonful of the powder of fried cumin seeds mixed with the pulp of a ripe banana can be taken just before going to sleep at night.

CIRRHOSIS OF THE LIVER
(Talaiff-ul-kabid)

When the healthy tissues of the liver become fibrous and scarred, it is called cirrhosis. The liver contracts in size. The first symptom of cirrhosis is loss of appetite; later, there is acute pain in the stomach where the liver is located. Among children it is faulty diet that gives rise to cirrhosis; among adults, it is generally due to too much alcohol.

Remedies
1. The best remedy for cirrhosis is *bhringaraja* (*Clerodendrum serratum*), a small marshland herb. A teaspoonful of the juice of this herb could be taken thrice a day with honey.
2. *Katuki* (*Picrorhiza kurroa*) is however the more popular drug for cirrhosis. One teaspoonful of the powder of the root of this herb should be mixed with honey and taken thrice every twenty-four hours.

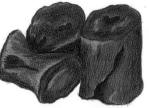

Rewand chini *or rhubarb. The root of this plant is very effective in avoiding cirrhosis of liver.*

Regimen
Drugs apart, the best remedy for cirrhosis is a diet free from fats and condiments and a complete avoidance of alcohol.

JAUNDICE *(Yarqan)*

Jaundice may be caused by an inflammation of the liver, obstruction of the bile ducts or even cirrhosis. The first symptoms of this disease is the appearance of an yellowish tinge in the whites of the eyes and the urine. In severe cases, even the skin turns yellow. If there is hepatitis (inflammation of the liver), there is usually pain in the region of the liver.

Remedies
1. The first and the foremost need in jaundice is to keep the patient on a restricted diet. All fats, spices and acidic substances should be avoided. As for medication, the drugs recommended for cirrhosis would help in case of jaundice too.

2. *Trivrit* (*Ipomoea-terpenthum*) and *katuki* may be powdered and two teaspoonfuls of this powder taken thrice a day with lukewarm water.
3. Twenty grams of *henna* leaves should be soaked in water overnight; the mixture should be strained in the morning and drunk for a few days.
4. Juice of the leaves of horse radish (10 gm) should be boiled, strained and drunk after 20 gm of raw sugar has been added to the mixture.

Regimen

The two main things to remember in case of jaundice is not to strain the liver (this could be ensured through regular and disciplined habits of excretion) and be on a fat free diet. The organ will then recover even without medication. Sweet substances and liquids like sugarcane juice, fruit juices and dry grapes should form the patient's diet. About 100 gm of dried tamarind (*imli*)

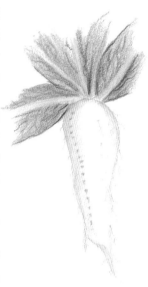

Turb *or radish, usually prescribed for those suffering from jaundice.*

should be soaked in water overnight with half the quantity of dried plums (*aloo bukhara*); and the thick liquid drunk by adding a little salt to it in the morning. The patient should drink plenty of water throughout the day.

HYPERTENSION
(Zaght-ud-dam qawi)

The normal blood pressure in a healthy adult is generally taken to be about 120 to 140 mm of mercury systolic (when the heart contracts) and 80 to 85 mm of mercury diastolic (when the heart expands). If the pressure rises beyond this range, there are symptoms like headache, a constant humming sound in the ears, insomnia, tachycardia, giddiness and a general feeling of weakness.

Remedies

The treatment of hypertension must start with a proper diagnosis of its origin. If it is secondary, i.e.

if it is caused by some other disease like nephritis or diabetes, treatment of that malady should be first undertaken. But if it is of primary origin, one should take garlic, one of the most effective natural drugs in controlling blood pressure. A paste made of one gram of garlic mixed with a glass of buttermilk or whey taken twice a day will help bring down the blood pressure. An alternate remedy for hypertension is the root of the drug *sarpagandha* (*Rauwolfia serpentina*) in a powdered form. Half a teaspoonful of this drug taken thrice a day deals with hypertension effectively.

HYPOTENSION
(*Zaght-ud-dam zaeef*)

Low blood pressure or hypotension may be caused by a haemorrhage owing to injury, bursting of an ulcer of the stomach or nose bleed. Food poisoning and anaemia may also lead to low blood pressure.

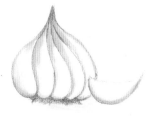

Seer *or garlic. A very effective natural drug for controlling high blood pressure, specially due to high levels of cholesterol.*

Remedies

If the pressure falls on account of an injury, the patient should be removed to the hospital and given a blood transfusion. If hypotension is caused by anaemia, it can be cured only when anaemia has been effectively dealt with. Brandy or alcohol of any variety in quantities from 15 to 50 ml diluted with warm water is a temporary cure which can be tried till the exact cause of the malady is ascertained.

Regimen

A patient suffering from low blood pressure should be advised to rest. The best diet for a hypotense patient is boiled vegetables and fruits. Strenuous exercise should be avoided but long walks in the morning and evening would help.

TACHYCARDIA OR PALPITATION
(*Khafkhaan*)

The heart beats at the rate of 72 to 80 beats per minute. But if the pulse rate goes beyond the normal range when an individual is not performing any physical exercise, the condition is known as tachycardia. A heavy stomach, flatulence and constipation are contributory factors in tachycardia and must be dealt with before treatment can start. If the patient is a smoker, he or she should give it up immediately.

Remedies

1. Equal amounts of aniseed, dry coriander and jaggery should be powdered and taken in six-gram doses after each meal.
2. Alternatively, five grams of aniseed, three grams of coriander and eleven pieces of raisins should be soaked in water or rose water overnight and this water strained and drunk every morning.

SCURVY (*Sakur-boot*)

In this condition, there is bleeding of the gums because of a lack of Vitamin C. This makes the capillaries

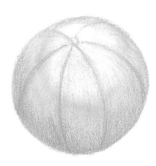

Amla *or emblic myrobalan, the richest source of Vitamin C and the best remedy for scurvy.*

fragile and ruptures them, leading to extensive haemorrhage and in extreme cases, formation of glandular patches similar to boils all over the body, particularly in the lower limbs.

Remedies

The only way to deal with scurvy is to take massive doses of Vitamin C. The best remedy is *amla*, probably the richest natural source of the vitamin. One teaspoonful of the powder of dried *amla* mixed with an equal amount of sugar should be taken thrice daily with milk. The patient's diet should be abundant in fresh fruits like oranges and guavas.

DYSURIA (*Usrat-ul-boul*)

Dysuria means difficulty or pain during urinating.

Remedies

1. Whatever the cause of retention of urine, 2 gm of a mixture of black mustard, nitre (1 gm each) and raw sugar taken with water

every two hours would definitely bring relief.

2. If urine has been retained for a long time, a piece of cloth soaked in a solution of nitre in water can be placed on the pelvis.

RENAL COLIC (Waja-ul-kuliya)

Renal colic is a condition in which there is pain in the kidneys. This occurs when a stone lodges itself in the ureter. The pain is agonising and shoots down from the kidney region to the groin and appears all of a sudden.

Remedies

Twenty grams of black cumin seeds, 10 gm of *ajwain* and 6 gm of black salt should be ground together and mixed with a little vinegar. This could be taken after adding 3 gm of ginger juice with a little asafoetida and a pinch of salt.

SCALDING URINE (Hirqat-ul-boul)

A burning sensation during urination may be due to hyperacidity or due

Khardal or black mustard seeds are very useful in treating painful micturition.

to some malfunctioning of the kidneys.

Remedies

1. A quarter litre of milk should be boiled with an equal quantity of water and drunk.

2. Alternatively, 10 gm each of nitre and a large cardamom should be ground together and the powder taken in four-gram doses with water or milk.

POLYURIA (Kasrat-ul-boul)

Polyuria, or excess of urine may be due to excessive intake of liquids or failure of the perspiration glands to function.

Remedies

1. Unripe pods of the acacia tree should be dried in the shade, fried and then powdered. Three grams of this powder taken in the morning and evening provides relief.

2. A medicinal concoction from

black sesame seeds can be prepared by taking 40 gm of the seeds, 20 gm of *ajwain* and 60 gm of jaggery and mixing them. Six grams of this mixture should be taken in the morning and evening. Polyuria of old age can be cured by this method.

3. Tamarind seeds and horse radish leaves should be ground together in lukewarm water and applied to the pelvic region.

4. Three grams of the powder of *kulanjan* taken with water also helps alleviating the condition.

BED-WETTING (*Boul-filfarash*)

Infants and young children tend to pass urine while sleeping.

Remedy

Twenty grams of sesame seeds should be mixed with 10 gm of *ajwain* and 30 gm of jaggery. Six grams of this concoction should be taken in the morning and evening.

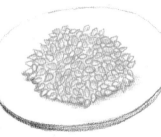

Kunjad or sesame seeds taken with food help in combating bed-wetting.

Regimen

A person susceptible to this disorder must empty his or her bladder before going to sleep.

AMENORRHOEA (*Ehtibas-ut-tams*)

Failure of menstruation to appear at all in a young woman may be due to anaemia, ill health and other diseases.

Remedies

1. A week before the menstrual period is due, a decoction of six grams of jaggery and twenty grams of clarified butter should be taken daily.

2. A mixture of carrot seeds and jaggery could be taken for about a week.

3. Another remedy is to soak 10 gm of black sesame seeds and an equal quantity of small caltrops in 250 ml of water, grind the seeds, add sugar to this mixture and drink it as a beverage.

DYSMENORRHOEA
(Usrat-ut-tams)

When cramps and pain in the groin precede the menstrual flow, they are signs of irritation in the ovaries.

Remedies

1. One hundred grams of the juice of the green leaves of black nightshade or *mako* (*Solanum nigrum*) and leaves of chicory or *kasni* (*Cichorium intibus*) should be warmed and when the mixture coagulates, it should be strained and drunk after adding 20 gm of jaggery to it.

2. A very effective remedy for the pain of dysmenorrhoea is a decoction of the root of the cotton tree (18 gm), *Bolus armenia rubra* or *telia geru* (6 gm), rose bush leaves (6 gm), the root of *Amaranthus paniculatus* or *chulai* (6 gm), jaggery (24 gm) boiled in 750 ml of water till one-eighth of it is left. This mixture

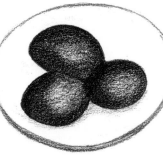

Mako or black nightshade. A useful anti-inflammatory drug.

should be taken for three days continuously during the menstrual period.

MENORRHAGIA (Kasrat-ut-tams)

If there is excessive discharge of blood during the monthly menstrual periods, it is called menorrhagia. Neglect of the condition or ineffective attempts at dealing with it may lead to anaemia of the most severe type.

Remedies

1. A home remedy is to grind seven pomegranate leaves and seven grains of rice into a paste and give it to the patient for a month twice daily.

2. Twenty grams of the bark of the *ashoka* (*Saraca indica*) tree should be crushed and boiled in 250 ml of milk and an equal amount of water. When half of the liquid is left, it should be strained, sweetened with sugar, and drunk. If this is taken for a

few days the patient will be on the road to recovery.

3. Half-ripe fruits of the country fig tree should be dried in the shade, powdered and mixed with an equal quantity of sugar. Six grams of the powder taken with milk in the morning and evening will give relief.

4. Three grams of *rasaut* and an equal quantity of *shellac* (*Laccifer lacca*) should be finely ground together and divided into two doses, one to be taken with milk in the morning and one in the evening.

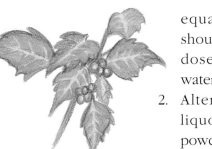

Rasaut *or Indian barberry. An effective drug to stop excessive blood flow in piles and menstruation.*

LEUCORRHOEA *(Sailan-ur-rahm)*

Leucorrhoea, also called whites, is a condition in which there is a white discharge from the vagina. A proper diagnosis of the causes of the malady should be made before treatment starts.

Remedies

1. The powdered bark of the *moolsari* tree mixed with an equal amount of raw sugar should be taken in nine-gram doses every morning with water.

2. Alternatively, dry *amla* and liquorice in equal quantities, powdered and mixed with thrice the quantity of honey is an effective drug for this disease.

FLACCIDITY OF THE BREASTS
(Takhalkhul-e-pistan)

The breasts have a tendency to sag and become flaccid with age. But in some cases this condition is manifested at a comparatively early age.

Remedies

1. Unripe fruits of the *moolsari* tree should be rubbed in water and applied over the breasts for eight to ten days.

2. Tender aerial roots of the banyan tree ground with a little water may be applied as a paste on the breasts for a week to ten days.

3. Another remedy is to grind the leaves of *chhumui* (*Mimosa pudica*) which is a type of the touch-me-not plant and the root of winter cherry or *asgand* (*Withania somnifera*) in water and apply the paste on the breasts for ten to twelve days.

THREATENED ABORTIONS
(Isqat-e-munazzrah)

If there is spotting during pregnancy, it may be a precursor to abortion and steps must be taken immediately. The patient must be advised to take rest and desist from heavy physical or mental work.

Remedies

1. The fruit of preserved *amla*, wrapped in silver foil should be eaten daily during the period of pregnancy.
2. Crushed white rose petals in ten to twenty-gram doses can be taken every day.

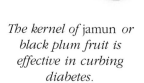

The kernel of jamun *or black plum fruit is effective in curbing diabetes.*

3. Unripe pods of acacia and leaf shoots of the banyan tree should be taken in equal quantities and dried in the shade. The powder of the two, mixed with an equal amount of raw sugar, taken in six gram-doses along with milk for a few days would deal with the danger of abortion.
4. Ten grams each of *amla, lodh pathani* (*Symplocos recemosus*) and liquorice should be finely ground mixed with an equal quantity of raw sugar. A six-gram dose every morning and evening will stop the bleeding.

DIABETES *(Ziabetes)*

Diabetes is a disease in the cure of which diet plays a more important part than drugs. It is vital therefore, that once the disease has been diagnosed and its severity ascertained from an examination of blood and urine that the diet of the patient be controlled. In this disease, the level of insulin, the hormone which controls amount of sugar in the blood goes down. Hence, blood sugar becomes high. The patient manifests this disease by urinating far too often, through swelling and pain in the feet.

Remedies

1. Seven leaves of *kanduri* (*Coccinia cordiofolia*) should be ground with seven grains of pepper, strained and drunk to reduce blood sugar.
2. Ten grams of *sankhaholi* (*Evolvulus alsinoides*) should also be ground with seven grains of pepper, strained and drunk.
3. Another useful remedy is 20 gm of the kernel of *jamun* (*Eugenia jambolana*) and 20 gm of poppy seeds ground together and taken in three gram-doses with whey or water every morning and evening.

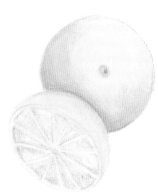

Limu *or lemon juice taken on an empty stomach helps in controlling obesity.*

OBESITY *(Siman-e-mufrat)*

The state of obesity can be loosely defined as an over-accumulation of fat in the body.

Remedies

1. The treatment of obesity must start with a severe restriction of the diet of the patient. Gum resin of the herb *guggulu* (*Commiphora mukul*) is the ideal drug for this condition. One gram of this powder should be taken four times a day with hot water.
2. Lemon juice and honey mixed with water taken first thing in the morning helps reduce excess fat.

Regimen

Regular jogging is the best exercise to reduce fat. Along with jogging, swimming and cycling everyday also help in combating obesity.

Glossary

— ❋ —

A

Afal-e-badam—Functions of the body.

Akhlat—Body fluids or humours. There are four according to Unani theory: blood, phlegm, yellow bile, black bile.

Al Havi Libre Continents—Text on the practical and clinical concepts of Unani medicine written by 10th century Arab scholar Rhazes.

Al Qanon Fit Tibb—The most famous book on Unani medicine written by the legendary Arab scholar Ibn Sina (AD 980-1037).

Al Tasreef—Ancient book on surgery written by 10th century Unani surgeon Zahravi.

Alamat—Symptoms of a disease.

Amal-e-kai—Cauterization, a surgical method in which direct heat is applied to the body mainly to remove unhealthy flesh.

Arkan—Basic elements which make up everything in the universe including the human body.

Arz—After-effects of a disease. Also, earth, one of the four primary elements.

Asb—Nerve

Asbab-e-badia—Causes of diseases which stem from external factors.

Asbab-e-batina—Causes of diseases which are internal in nature.

Asbab-e-marz—Causes of diseases.

Asbab-e-sittah zaruriah—The six essential factors responsible for maintaining good health in an individual. These are—air, food and drink, bodily movement and repose, mental movement and repose, sleeping habits, activities of retention and excretion.

Azah—Organs of the body which constitute its solid part.

Azah-e-damwiah—Organs which are formed in the foetal stage from the mother's blood.

Azah-e-manwiah—Organs which according to Unani theory originate from the semen when the foetus is being formed.

Azah-e-raisah—Vital organs on which the essential powers of the body depend.

Azm—Bone

B

Bahut-e-saut—Hoarseness of the voice

Balgam—Phlegm, one of the four humours.

Balghami mizaj—A phlegmatic temperament in which phlegm predominates amongst the four humours.

Baraz—Foecal matter

Barid—Cold

Bars—Leucoderma

Boul—Urine

Boul-filfarash—Bed-wetting

C

Chini tibb—Medicine which developed in the ancient Chinese civilization.

D

Dalak—Massage

Dam—Blood, one of the four humours which determine the state of the body.

Damwi mizaj—A sanguine temperament in which the qualities of blood predominate.

Dimagh—The brain, one of the essential organs of the body.

Dumbul and nifaat—Boils and pustules

E

Ehtibas—Retention of digested matter in the body.

Ehtibas-ut-tams—Amenorrhoea or failure of menstruation to occur at all.

F

Fasd—Venesection, a surgical method in which a vein is cut open to shed impure blood.

Fovaque—Hiccup

G

Ghee—A type of clarified liquid butter used widely in India both as a cooking base and for general consumption.

Ghishah—Membrane

Ghiza-e-lateef—Liquid diet

Ghiza-e-mutadil—Normal diet

Ghiza-e-mutawassat—Semi-solid diet

Ghuzruf—Cartilage

H

Hamman—Steam bath

Har—Wet

Harkat—Movement

Hasaf—Prickly heat

Hawah—Air, one of the four primary elements.

Hifzan-e-sehat —Hygiene

Hijamat—Cupping, a surgical method in which excess quantity of humours is removed.

Hindi tibb—Indian medicine

Hirqat-ul-boul—Scalding urine

Humma-e-umoomi—Fever

Huqnah—Enema, a type of regimental therapy.

Husra—Constipation

I

Inhetat—The stage of retardation when a disease starts to decelerate.

Ibtida—The beginning or onset of a disease.

Ifrat-e-ghiza—Precribing excess food, a practice in diet-o-therapy.

Ilaj-biddawah—Pharmacotherapy, one of the four major Unani therapies. In this, drugs of natural origin are prescribed.

Ilaj-bil-ghiza—Diet-o-therapy, also one of the four major Unani therapies. In this, alterations in the patient's diet are suggested.

Ilaj-bit-tadbir—Regimental therapy, one of the four therapies. In this no drugs are prescribed and certain regimens like exercise, massage and steam baths are suggested which aim at minimum invasion of the patient's body.

Ilmul-amaraaz—Pathology, in Unani medicinal parlance.

Imtizaj haquiqui—When a new compound with qualities which resemble nothing of its constituent elements is formed.

Intaha—The stage of saturation when a disease is at its peak.

Ishaal—Purging toxic waste matter through the bowels, a type of regimental theapy. Also diarrhoea.

Isqat-e-munazzrah—Spotting during pregnancy.

Istafraagh—Excretion of undigested matter.

J

Jarhat—Surgery, also one of the four therapies. In this, specialized surgical methods such as venesection, leeching, diathermy etc. are used.

K

Kabid—The liver, one of the essential organs.

Kasrat-ul-boul—Polyuria

Kasrat-ut-tams—Menorrhagia or excessive discharge of blood during menstruation.

Khafkhaan—Tachycardia

Khilafat-e-abbasia—The golden period of the Arab civilization (AD 749-1258). This period includes the rule of famous Arab king Haroon Rashid.

Khisya—The testes, also one of the essential organs.

Kirm-e-shikam—Intestinal parasites

L

Lahem—Flesh

M

Ma—Water, one of the four primary elements.

Makool—Food

Mani—Semen

Marz—Disease

Mashroob—Substances which can be drunk i.e water, milk, tea, alcohol.

Misri Tibb—Ancient Egyptian medicine

Mizaj—Temperament which is determined by the way primary elements combine in a substance.

Mizaj-e-ghair mutadil—Unequal temperament or the temperament of a compound in which the contrary qualities of constituent elements are unbalanced.

Mizaj-e-mutadil—Equal temperament or the temperament of a compound in which the contrary qualities of constituent elements are perfectly balanced.

Mufrad—Simple

Muhazzil—Weight-reducing drugs

Mukkh—Bone marrow

Murakkab—Compound

N

Nabz—Pulse

Nafakh—Flatulence

Nar—Fire, one of the four primary elements.

Nar-e-faarsi—Eczema

Naum—State in which an individual is awake.

Nazla-e-wabaiyah—Influenza

Q

Qae—Emesis, a type of regimental therapy.

Qalb—The heart, one of the essential organs of the body.

Quwat—Faculty or phenomenon by which all life functions are manifested in an individual.

Quwat-e-haiwaniya—Vital or physical faculty

Quwat-e-nafsaniya—Mental faculty

Quwat-e-tabia—Natural faculty

R

Ramad—Conjunctivitis

Ratab—Wet

Riyazat—Exercise

Rooh—Gaseous, also refers to oxygen which is considered vital air.

Ruaaf—Nose bleed

S

Saafah—Baldness

Sabab—A specific disturbance which brings about a change in the body either from sickness to health or vice versa.

Safra—Yellow bile, one of the four humours.

Safravi mizaj—A bilious temperament in which yellow bile predominates.

Sahar—Insomnia

Sailan-ur-rahm—Leucorrhoea or white discharge from the vagina.

Sakur-boot—Scurvy

Sauda—Black bile, one of the four humours.

Saudavi mazaj—A melancholic temperament in which black bile predominates.

Shaeb-e-shaar—Premature greying

Shaeirah—Stye

Shahem—Fat

Shahiquah—Whooping cough

Shar—Hair

Shara—Urticaria

Shiryan—Artery

Siman-e-mufrat—Obesity

Suaal—Cough

Sue mizaj—Abnormal temperament Here, diseases which are caused by an imbalance in the humours.

Sue tarkeeb—Abnormal structure. Here, diseases which are caused by malformations in the body.

Sukoon nafsania—A state in which the mind is relaxed and rested.

Sum—Literally, poison. In this case, drugs which act so fast on the body that they can have toxic effects.

Susruta Samhita—One of the most authoritative Ayurvedic texts written by ancient Hindu sage Susruta.

T

Ta farruque wa ittisaal—Abnormal discontinuity or adhesion. Here, diseases which result due to injuries and abnormal healing.

Tabdeel-e-ghiza—Alterations in a patient's diet which are done in various ways as a part of diet-o-therapy.

Tabiat—According to Unani theory, a divine power given to every individual by nature for sustenance of health.

Tabiatul Insan—Book by legendary Greek healer Hippocrates (460-377 BC).

Takhahalkhul-e-pistan—Flaccidity of the breasts.

Talaiff-ul-kabid—Cirrhosis of the liver.

Taleeque—Leeching, an ancient method of surgery in which infected blood is removed from the body with the help of leeches.

Tamkeed—Fomentation, a type of regimental therapy.

Tanasur-wa-tamrat—Patchy baldness

Tark-e-ghiza—Prohibition of food, a method used in diet-o-therapy.

Tazaiyud—The stage at which a disease accelerates.

Tiryan-ud-dum-lissah—Loose and bleeding teeth.

Tukhma—Dyspepsia

U

Umure tabaiyah—The concept of the body under Unani physiology.

Unani tibb—Medicine which originated in ancient Greece and was expanded and improvised in 8th-13th century Arabia.

Usrat-ul-boul—Dysuria or pain while urinating.

Usrat-ut-tams—Dysmenorrhoea or painful menstruation.

V

Vaidyas—Ayurvedic doctors

W

Waja-ul-kuliya—Renal colic

Wajaul-asnaan—Toothache

Warid—Vein

Warm-e-lauzatain—Tonsillitis

Warm-e-shob—Bronchitis and bronchial asthma

Wat'r—Tendon

Y

Yabis—Dry

Yaqzah—Sleep

Yarqan—Jaundice

Z

Zaght-ud-dam-qawi—Hypertension

Zaght-ud-dam-zaeef—Hypotension

Zaheer—Dysentery

Zeequn-nafas—Asthma

Ziabetes—Diabetes

Zufur—Nail